Understanding and Tackling Obesity

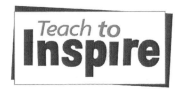

www.teachingexpertise.com/teachtoinspire

Understanding and Tackling Obesity:
A Whole School Programme

Ruth MacConville

Author:
Ruth MacConville

Designer:
Jess Wright
Cover image: ©istockphoto.com/ Kameleon007

Editor:
George Robinson

Copy Editor:
Mel Maines

Illustrator:
Andrew Chubb (Andrew_Chubb@sky.com)

007-5823/Printed in the United Kingdom by CMP

Published by Speechmark Publishing Ltd., Unit C5, Sunningdale House, 43 Caldecotte Lake Drive, Caldecotte Lake Business Park, Milton Keynes, Bucks, MK7 8LF, UK

www.speechmark.net

British Library Cataloguing in Publication Data

A catalogue record for this book is available from the British Library

ISBN 978-1-906517-58-8

A CD-ROM is attached to the inside front cover and is an integral part of this publication.

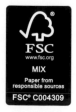

Contents

Acknowledgements   3

Part One: Setting the Scene   5

Introduction   7

Part Two: Staff Preparation   43

PowerPoint Presentation   45

General Guidance on Delivering the Programme   69

Guidance on Practical Aspects of Delivering the Programme   73

Working with Parents   78

Part Three: Happy, Healthy You Programme   85

Session 1: Happy, Healthy You   87

Session 2: High Five Foods   105

Session 3: What to Eat?   113

Session 4: Full   119

Session 5: How to Read Food Labels   125

Session 6: Healthy Snacks   131

Session 7: Get Moving   137

Session 8: Get Moving Some More   143

Session 9: TV Turnoff   149

Session 10: Media Messages   155

Session 11: Everybody's Different   161

Session 12: Let's Celebrate   167

Part Four   171

Useful Websites and Further Reading   173

References   177

Use of the CD-ROM

Many Teach to Inspire publications include CD-ROMs to support the purchaser in the delivery of the training or teaching activities. These may include any of the following file formats:

- PDFs requiring Acrobat v.3.
- Microsoft Word files.
- Microsoft PowerPoint files.
- Video clips which can be played by Windows Media Player.
- If games are included the software required is provided on the CD-ROM.

All material on the accompanying CD-ROM can be printed by the purchaser/user of the book. This includes library copies. Some of this material is also printed in the book and can be photocopied but this will restrict it to the black and white/greyscale version when there might be a colour version on the CD-ROM.

The CD-ROM itself must not be reproduced or copied in its entirety for use by others without permission from the publisher.

All material on the CD-ROM is © MacConville 2012

Website addresses are correct at the time the book is proofed for publication. Unfortunately site owners do make frequent changes. If an address does not lead effectively to the required site we would advise you to do a search using the significant words in the www address.

Symbol Key

 This symbol indicates a page that can be photocopied from the book or printed from the PDF file on the CD-ROM. The book title appears on the page in the book but not on copies printed from the CD-ROM.

 This symbol indicates a page that can be photocopied from the book or modified and printed from the Word file on the CD-ROM. The book title appears on the page in the book but not on copies printed from the CD-ROM.

Dedication: For Andrew, Matthew and Yvonne, as always.

Acknowledgements

This book would not have been written without the contributions of the children and young people who have shared with me their stories, thoughts and feelings and have taught me so much.

I would also like to thank the many parents and practitioners I have worked with over the years and from whom I have learned so much.

Special thanks to my colleagues Eulalee Green and Michelle Wakeley both of whom are HPC registered dieticians and have provided much encouragement and many helpful conversations throughout the process of writing this book. Special thanks also to my colleague Karen Gibson, Health Improvement Advisor, for her encouragement and for creating many helpful and enjoyable opportunities to share thoughts and ideas.

I would like to thank my wonderful editors George Robinson and the late Barbara Maines who believed in this book since its inception. Special thanks to George who has always been available for helpful advice and has provided invaluable encouragement.

Finally, a tremendous thanks to family and friends for their patience during periods of hibernation while I worked on this book.

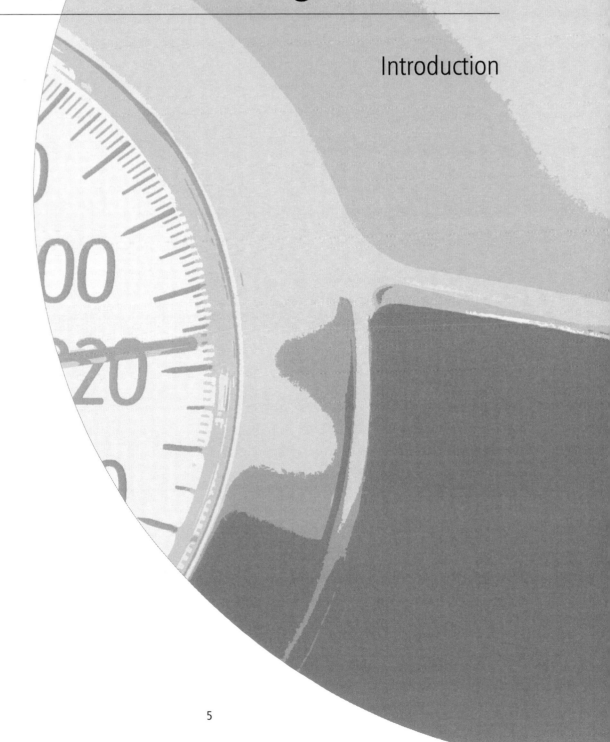

Part One: Setting the Scene

Introduction

Introduction

Welcome to this book. For those readers who want to start to find out immediately about delivering the programme that forms the backbone of this book, please turn to Part Three. For those readers who want to know more about the theory behind the programme and the context of this book, read on.

In England, more than 60 per cent of adults and 30 per cent of children are either overweight or obese. We are now officially the fattest nation in Europe (Malholtra, 2011). Almost daily, headlines in the national press draw our attention to debilitating eating disorders and a rise in childhood obesity. These problems are triggered by society's preoccupation with the thin ideal and the multiple, conflicting messages that promote unhealthy attitudes and behaviours. From a very early age, children are bombarded with messages from food manufacturers to consume their products that are often full of saturated fats, sugars and salt. These messages have an especially negative effect as children experience the natural reshaping of their bodies during puberty. Skilful advertising makes these 'foods' seem fun, cool, delicious and even empowering and seeks to engage the young person's sense of self-esteem. Excessive consumption of these products, however, inevitably leads to poor health as they are often addictive and by the time children reach the age at which they can reasonably be expected to make their own choices, many of them are already hooked. Body image, eating, fitness, nutrition and weight problems are pervasive in our culture and many children today are reported to be worried about their size, shape and weight. These concerns diminish children's self-esteem and confidence as well as demanding the attention and energy that should be available for more important developmental tasks. It is well documented that body-angst, eating, fitness and weight problems are very difficult to reverse once they are established. Early interventions are, therefore, needed to target the context within which the variety of body image, eating, nutrition, fitness and weight problems multiply. This book explores a strengths approach to enabling children to develop positive living skills. The most fundamental way in which we can do this, is by demonstrating a positive, healthy outlook on life ourselves and by committing ourselves to discovering our own strengths and the strengths of others.

The programme, 'Happy, Healthy You', which is presented in Part Three of this book has been designed to proactively teach children that health, not size or shape, is a reliable reward for healthy choices and that self-respect, body esteem as well as nutritional health and physical fitness are achievable for all children at every size. It focuses on expanding pupils' self-identity and sense of self-worth, thus decreasing the emphasis and importance of physical appearance. A strong message of the programme is that everybody's different and nobody is perfect. This approach to health is realistic and non-discriminatory and aims to enable children, from an early age, to recognise and resist unhealthy pressures, maintain body esteem and know how to make skilled choices that will ensure their health and wellbeing.

Using this Book

This book is written in four parts that interlock like a jigsaw. Following this opening, the next section contains an introduction to the ideas on which the programme is based. Teachers are advised to read this section to become familiar with the concepts that the programme teaches and also in order to understand its approach. This background section should be made available to all staff to ensure that there is a consistent set of messages about positive living skills throughout the school.

The second part of the book contains a PowerPoint presentation that can be used to introduce the programme to staff. It contains background information on positive living skills and an overview of the sessions. This is followed by a section that offers practical guidance on how to deliver the programme.

The third part contains the facilitator notes and the 12 sessions.

The book ends with suggestions for further reading and a list of useful websites.

About the Programme

Happy, Healthy You is a stand-alone programme that aims to increase children's wellbeing by equipping them with the knowledge and skills that they need to lead healthy and happy lives. The programme focuses on positive living skills that will not only help pupils to be healthier and happier right now, but will also provide the knowledge and skills that they need for lifelong health. Healthy living encompasses more than just eating a nutritious and balanced diet. It involves getting the exercise and rest our bodies need to stay healthy, as well as engaging in activities that we enjoy and that enhance our mental and social wellbeing.

Throughout the programme a range of self-reflection activities have been designed to enable pupils to develop healthy eating habits, increase their physical activity and limit screen time while at the same time building skills in personal, health and social domains. The programme encourages pupils to think about how healthy living and wellness makes everything else, including learning and making friends, happen. Spending time with friends can provide support for the many challenges we face in life, as well as provide companions for physical activity. The key to healthy living is a balance of all aspects of life to include the physical, intellectual, social and emotional.

The programme aims to teach pupils the practical skills that they can use to make their lives go better through a developmental programme of action. The sessions are interactive and largely based on group discussions and partner work to ensure that pupils learn more about themselves and others. They should be delivered with a sense of fun in order to engage and inspire all learners.

The programme uses an interactive approach to teaching and learning. This approach emphasises that individuals learn best when they actively construct meaning for themselves. Pupils come to school with a diverse range of knowledge and experiences and it is important that this knowledge is celebrated. The programme has been designed to encourage teachers to create learning environments that recognise and build on this diversity in a way that is active, inquiry based, and pupil centred.

The programme consists of 12 sessions. Each session starts by activating and reviewing pupils' prior knowledge. Sessions continue with inquiry-based activities that aim to engage children in critical thinking in addition to building new skills. Every session provides ideas for whole-class discussions and suggestions for small group and partner work to enable pupils to explore health-related issues. Social development is enhanced throughout the programme by the opportunities that children have to work cooperatively with each other.

The programme is suitable for pupils throughout the primary phase, with the expectation that teachers will adapt it to suit the range of abilities and learning styles. Its content has been found to be highly appealing to pupils with a range of abilities, learning styles and personalities. The sessions have been designed to be delivered in sequence to maximise and reinforce learning.

Pupils are encouraged to practise the skills and ideas that are introduced in the sessions in their day-to-day lives with home practice in the form of 'take away' activities that are a core element of the programme.

Throughout the programme, pupils are taught how to initiate change in their lives in order to become healthier and more resilient. Samuel Smiles, father of the modern self-help movement (quoted in Ben-Shahar, 2007), wrote:

> Every youth should be made to feel that his well doing in life must necessarily rely mainly on himself and the exercise of his own energies, rather than upon the help and patronage of others.

Understanding Obesity

Do we say overweight, obese or fat?

'Obese' from the Latin word 'obesus' means 'grown fat by eating'. The term's origin suggests that overeating is a major cause of the obesity epidemic. Teaching overweight children to eat less is essential. However, modifying behaviour is no simple task and eating too much is not the sole cause of obesity. Other factors play a role and must be understood in order to reverse the epidemic and produce healthier generations of children.

Sharron Dalton (2004) writes that health professionals and the media have been doing 'an interesting dance' around the term 'obesity'. They use it freely in the abstract and in reference to the general population, but they apply it with caution when describing individuals, especially children. 'Overweight' has developed into a more acceptable and sensitive synonym for 'obese'. In the UK both of the 'O' words, however, are considered more acceptable and more polite than the F-word, fat. A notable exception to this rule recently hit the headlines when Georgia Davis, a 17 year old from South Wales, was described as 'Britain's fattest teenager' weighing 40 stone and 6lb (*The Sunday Times*, 27.2.11).

Fat Studies

In the US where obesity in both children and adults is even more prevalent than in the UK, there is agreement in the radical, new academic field of Fat Studies that the 'O' words are neither neutral or kind. There is support for reclaiming the word 'fat' as a neutral adjective and as the preferred term of political identity. Rothblum and Solovay (2009) emphasise that the term fat is simply a descriptive term. Weight, like height, they suggest is a human characteristic that varies across any population like a bell curve. There have always been people of different heights and there will always be people of different weights. Fat Studies offer no opposition to what they regard as this simple fact of weight diversity. Throughout this book I use both terms 'overweight' and 'obese' interchangeably, as they are found in scientific and popular literature. In terms of working with individuals, I agree with Dalton (2004) that it is important to emphasise a 'healthy weight for you' as a positive way to talk about body size and health.

Prevalence

The Association for the Study of Obesity (2011) confirms that childhood obesity is a serious problem with profound health and social consequences. It has received substantial media attention recently, partly due to the rapid increase in occurrence across the UK, as well as internationally. This rise began to occur in the UK in the mid 1980s with a rapid increase most noticeably over the following ten years. The Health Survey for England (2007) reported that in the UK, obesity rose from 11 per cent of boys and 12 per cent of girls in 1995 to 17 per cent of boys and 16per cent of girls in 2007. Prevalence of obesity is even higher than that of the general population in some sub-groups of children including:

- survivors of many childhood cancers
- those living in socio-economically deprived families
- children from some minority ethnic groups
- children who are looked after
- those with at least one obese parent
- children and adolescents with learning difficulties.

    (NCB, 2011)

Current statistics suggest that the trend in obesity now appears to be flattening out. However, it will be important to continue to monitor the trends in future to confirm that this is a continuing pattern, or a plateau within a longer-term trend that is gradually increasing.

How Do We Know if a Child is Overweight or Obese?

Just looking at a child is not enough to determine whether they are overweight or obese. Smith (2008) writes that judgements made by teachers, parents and health professionals are often incorrect. Many adults don't recognise when there's a problem because so many children are now overweight and as a result what's considered to be the norm has changed. It is important, therefore, that a child's weight, in relation to their growth, is measured and interpreted appropriately. Childhood overweight and obesity can be diagnosed using the body mass index (BMI), but interpreting BMI in children is more complex than in adults. As children grow, BMI changes with age and there are differences between girls and boys, so it isn't possible to use single cut off points to denote overweight and obesity as they can for adults. Gender specific BMI charts are available from www.healthforallchildren. co.uk and can be used to determine and interpret BMI in children. The charts give two approaches to diagnosing obesity in children under the age of 18 years:

1. BMI above the 98th percentile for sex and age, recommended by the recent Scottish Intercollegiate Guidelines Network (SIGN), which published an evidence-based guideline for childhood obesity management (www.sign.ac.uk).

2. BMI above the 'international' definition (shown as the green obesity dotted line) provided by the International Obesity Task Force (IOTF).

Both of these definitions of obesity are cautious and conservative. They are highly specific for obesity with very low false positive rates, meaning that almost all children diagnosed as obese using BMI will be excessively fat and therefore at increased health risk.

For clinical purposes overweight can be defined as a BMI above the 91st percentile on the UK 1990 BMI charts or, alternatively, BMI above the dotted green line described as IOTF overweight.

The Consequences of Childhood Obesity

The Association for the Study of Obesity (2011) confirms that obesity in childhood is associated with numerous health and social consequences. These consequences are summarised below and can be divided into those that have an influence on short-term health and those that have longer-term outcomes.

Short-Term Consequences

Probably the most widespread consequence of overweight and obesity in children is psychological ill health. Social and psychological consequences can include stigmatisation, discrimination and prejudice. The extent to which obesity influences self-esteem seems to vary from one child to another, although there are suggestions that obese adolescents may be more affected than younger children. It is a complex issue but obesity in children has been linked to:

- low self-image
- low self-confidence
- depression.

The processes that lead to cardiovascular disease in adulthood are strongly associated with childhood obesity. The cardiovascular risk factors that have been identified include:

- raised blood lipids (fats) and insulin levels
- high blood pressure
- abnormalities in the size and function of the left ventricular mass (an indicator of the efficiency with which the heart pumps blood around the body).

The Association for the Study of Obesity (2011) estimates that two thirds of children of primary school age who are obese will have at least one of these cardiovascular risk factors, and approximately one-quarter will have two or more. Childhood obesity is also associated with increased risk of asthma and exacerbation of existing asthma and less frequently, sleep disorders, various joint problems and development of a fatty liver.

Longer-Term Consequences

There is a marked increase in the risk of ill health in adulthood that arises from obesity of childhood, independent of adult weight. The main risk is the persistence of obesity from childhood and adolescence to adulthood. Obese children are highly likely to become obese adults. It is estimated that 83 per cent of obese children aged 10 to 14 remain obese into adulthood (Department of Health, 2004). For adolescents and young adults who are obese there is an increased risk of lower educational attainment, social isolation and low income.

The overall effect is an increased risk of ill health and risk of premature death in adult life.

The severity of these consequences for both physical and mental health, highlight the importance of preventing obesity in children and adolescents as part of a comprehensive approach to tackling the obesity epidemic. Our weight is determined by how much exercise we take and by how much we eat. The Landmark Report for the Children's Society, *A Good Childhood* (Layard and Dunn, 2009), suggests that the most striking factor in recent years has been the decline in exercise. For children there have been three huge changes over the last fifty years:

1. Fewer children walk or bicycle to school (Dept of Health, 2004).

2. Children play less sport.

3. Children spend more time sitting in front of the television, computer or Playstation, rather than running around.

This trend reflects a move from active to passive leisure, which is undesirable, as our bodies and our minds both need physical exercise.

The programme is not about dieting or weight control. Jenny O' Dea (2007) writes that 'dietary restraint' during childhood and adolescence can have devastating effects on growth and development. Solovay (2000) confirms that when children are put on diets, there is evidence to suggest that their ability to recognise satiety may never develop or recover. It is therefore essential that teachers refrain from talking to pupils about weight loss and dieting. Kathy Kater (2005), a psychotherapist who has treated body image, eating, fitness and weight problems for more that two decades, emphasises that by now it should be clear to all that the identification of fatness as the problem and the resulting emphasis on weight loss as the solution has done little to address the health concerns of the next generation of children and, in fact, is making things worse. This mindset encourages the drive to be thin and the diet mentality, but has very little positive effect on the eating patterns, fitness or weight of the average child or adult. Kater writes:

> When we shift the focus from fat and weight to healthy choices leading to nutritional health and fitness, we sacrifice nothing and gain an approach that enhances the wellbeing of all.

Putting the positive living messages into practice can help everyone, both children and adults, improve their current wellbeing and decrease their risks for many chronic conditions and diseases. The practical experiences that adults have in putting the messages into practice for themselves and their family and friends, can be helpful in the process of guiding pupils through the programme. It is important when talking to pupils to emphasise the benefits of a healthy life style and avoid conveying an attitude of restriction. Pupils do not need to give up high-sugar foods or eliminate TV altogether.

Moderation is the Key

Sharron Dalton (2004), Professor in the Department of Nutrition, Food Studies and Public Health at New York University, writes that children can achieve a healthy weight through moderation. This involves measured behaviour in eating and physical activity patterns, rather than an overindulgence in portion sizes or an underestimation of the importance of daily physical activity. It also involves reasonable expectations about body sizes and shapes. It does not envisage a perfect diet, a perfect lifestyle, or a perfect body size. Aristotle's ancient wisdom still prevails that, 'as a general principle, moderation is always best'. The programme encourages pupils to think about their choices for nutrition and activity and gives them practice in developing a variety of practical and effective strategies for becoming healthier.

An Asset Approach

This book adopts an asset approach to building pupils' positive living skills. This approach values the capacity, skills, knowledge, connections and potential that exists in a community, in this case the school. Since the publication of the reports Glass Half Full (Foot and Hopkins, 2010) and What Makes Us Healthy? (Foot, 2012) interest in asset-based working has mushroomed and found its way into reports, guidance and research on the future of public health, social care and wellbeing. A growing body of evidence shows that when practitioners begin with a focus on what communities have, that is, their assets, as opposed to what they don't have, their needs, an individual or a community's efficacy in addressing their own needs, increases.

The more familiar 'deficit' approach, on the other hand, focuses on problems, needs and deficiencies and designs interventions to fill the gaps and fix the problems. As a result individuals can feel dependent and passive. An asset approach enables individuals to be proactive in their own lives.

The shift from using a deficit to an asset based approach requires a change in attitudes and values. An asset approach values the capacity, skills, knowledge, connections and potential in a community. It is about celebrating pupils' existing practical skills and knowledge of positive living, their interests and networks and relationships. It doesn't only see the problems and gaps that need filling. The more familiar 'deficit' approach focuses on the problems, needs and health-damaging behaviours of individuals.

The asset approach is a set of values and principles and a way of thinking about the world. The approach:

- identifies and makes visible the health enhancing assets and behaviours in a community
- sees individuals as co-producers of health and wellbeing
- promotes relationships and friendships that can provide caring, mutual help and fun
- supports individuals health and wellbeing through building self-esteem, coping strategies, resilience, relationships, friendships, knowledge and personal resources.

An asset approach starts by asking questions and reflecting on what 'assets' are already in place:

- What makes us strong?
- What makes us healthy?
- What helps us cope when things get difficult?
- What makes this a good place to be?
- What can we do to improve our health?

In practice this means:

- finding out what is already working and generating more of it
- promoting more of what the programme is trying to achieve rather than focusing on what the problems are
- valuing the assets, as soon as individuals are talking to each other they are working on the solutions

- actively building confidence among pupils and staff
- involving all the individuals from the beginning as those left out will be left behind
- ensuring the long-term sustainability of the project.

Positive Psychology

An asset approach has a great deal in common with positive psychology. Positive psychology was officially launched as a field of study in 1998 by Martin Seligman. An important goal for positive psychology is advancing knowledge about how to help individuals increase their:

- level of happiness
- positive mental health
- personal thriving.

It brings scientific tools to the study of human flourishing. Felicia Huppert (2007) writes that it was previously assumed that the absence of human adversities would result in human flourishing. If poor physical health caused unhappiness then good physical health would result in human flourishing. Positive psychologists have discovered that strengths have their own patterns. The absence of illness is not a sufficient criterion for health, and flourishing is much more than the absence of misery.

This books draws on a number of key concepts from positive psychology. As Sonja Lyubomirsky (2007) discovered, each individual has a setpoint or characteristic level of happiness that is genetically determined and accounts for approximately 50per cent of each individual's happiness quota. According to this idea we all, inevitably, return to our individual setpoint following disruptive events, be they positive or negative. The happiness setpoint theory is similar to what experts have discovered about weight control. The weight setpoint theory says that people have a certain weight that is determined by gene metabolism and others factors and is difficult to change. You might lose weight or gain weight, but the body's natural tendency is to revert to your weight setpoint. With the correct sustained nutrition and exercise it is possible to move one's weight setpoint down within certain parameters, and similarly with our setpoint of happiness, it is possible to train ourselves to become happier. Seligman (2011) calls this 'learned optimism'.

Throughout the programme two key concepts from positive psychology, flow and savouring, are emphasised as being essential strategies for encouraging children to recognise that there is so much more to life than how they look.

The Silver Lining Behind the Cloud of Bad News

Taking a positive approach to the teaching of positive living skills is important. As Dalton (2004) emphasises, there is a silver lining behind the cloud of bad news about childhood obesity because while it is the most prevalent health affliction in children, it is also the most preventable, even though there is no magic bullet in the form of a pill or a solution in terms of government action. *A Good Childhood* (Layard and Dunn, 2009) states that the government's policy to reduce obesity in children is to provide information, to make healthy choices easier and to legislate only if all else fails. In 2004 the government was spending £7 million a year on advertising in favour of healthy eating, while the food industry was spending £743 million on advertising, in favour of unhealthy eating

(ONS, 2007). So far, little has happened to improve spending patterns and there is every indication that the problem will become more serious.

The good news is, however, that there are many steps that we can take individually and together as a community to combat this epidemic.

The first step is to celebrate that food in Britain today is more plentiful, more nutritious, more varied and more affordable than ever before. Scientific journalists Gary Taubes (2011) and Rob Lyons (2011) invite us to take a humane and rational view on how to approach food:

> Things have never been so good, let us relax and enjoy our good fortune while striving both to make things even better here and to make sure everyone in the world can take a seat at the feast.
>
> (Lyons, 2011)

Lyons (2011) identifies that one of the myths of the current food debate is that there was a Golden Age in which everyone ate well, with lots of locally produced meat, fruit and vegetables, lovingly prepared at home. This idyll is presented in sharp contrast to the modern way of eating which is based on fast foods, ready meals and 'junk foods'. Our children allegedly grow up on sweets and crisps, and wouldn't recognise a real vegetable if it bit them. Lyons suggests that both sides of this image are exaggerated. The reality is that the working classes in Britain did not eat well until comparatively recently. Food was expensive relative to people's income, and what they could afford was often monotonous and dull. Lyons reminds us that it is only with rising living standards, falling food prices and the appearance of supermarkets that a wide range of food is now available at affordable prices to the majority.

A Historical Perspective

Lyons (2011) suggests that what we need is a historical perspective. When we look back we can see how far we have come and how much better off we are now than in the past. The gains of the past should give us great confidence about humanity's capacity to cope with the challenges of the future. There are reasons to be confident:

- There are rules imposed on every part of the food chain to ensure high standards.
- Our food is safe and we know that from our own experience.
- The supermarket chains have a material interest in maintaining a good reputation.

Thus a powerful mixture of trust and accountability makes buying food reassuringly predictable. Lyons suggests that 'a large side order of faith in the people around us would allow us to enjoy our food in peace'.

Balance, Variety and Moderation

In terms of teaching children about healthy eating habits there is also plenty to celebrate. Food and nutrition are interesting and relevant topics and rather than focusing on telling children what not to eat, the emphasis should be on encouraging them to enjoy healthy options. O'Dea (2007) suggests that the key components of healthy, human nutrition are:

- balance
- variety

- moderation.

There is no one food that cannot be included in a balanced diet. Lyons (2011) suggests that one of our 'societal eating problems' is to categorise food into good and bad. However, what is categorised as 'junk food' is often more nutritious than that which is regarded as wholesome. Stanley Feldman (2005) notes in his book *Panic Nation* that the term 'junk food' is an oxymoron. Either something is a food, in which case it is not junk, or it has no nutritional value, in which case it cannot be called a food. It is important when talking about food and nutrition to children to keep the focus positive, rather than negative, critical or blaming. Teachers and parents should avoid talking about 'good' and 'bad' foods or using the term 'junk food' as it is likely to create blame and guilt. It is also likely to make 'bad' foods more desirable. Jenny O'Dea (2007) suggests that it is not surprising that many young people choose to 'pig out' on 'forbidden' foods like cakes, biscuits, ice cream and chocolate.

Taking a positive, practical food-orientated approach is vital to helping children build healthy eating habits. This approach should include the preparation and enjoyment of quick and simple healthy meals and snacks. Talking about food is far more realistic and meaningful than talking about nutrients. Another aspect of teaching nutrition in a positive way is exploring with pupils about food in other cultures and celebrating the diversity of foods and recipes.

Savouring

Positive emotion in the present means experiencing good feelings in the 'here and now'. Positive psychologists suggest that we are often too busy planning what we are going to do next to really pay attention to the present. It is not too difficult to see how not paying attention to food when we are eating, may encourage us to eat more than we need, which is an important message with the current epidemic of obesity.

We can learn how to maximise pleasure in our life if we learn techniques to enhance savouring. So, for example, if we really enjoy eating a particular food, rather than encountering this pleasure every day, it may be beneficial to keep the pleasure for special occasions and not undermine it by too frequent use. Fred Bryant and Joseph Veroff (2007) have undertaken extensive research with children and young people on what enhances pleasure. Some of their techniques include involving children in discussions about:

- the types of food they find pleasurable and how much they pay attention to what they are eating

- ways that they can enhance their experience of pleasure, for example, through being involved with others. This is why eating with others is much more satisfying than eating alone.

Encouraging children to savour their food and give it their full and undivided attention will deepen their awareness and enjoyment of food. Introduce children to savouring by eating something delicious together as a class. This is an activity that is usually very well received. Encourage children to take every step slowly while focusing on what they are doing:

- Take a small piece of everyday food.

- Take your time to notice everything about it.

- Look at the shape and the colour.

- Notice its aroma.
- Then slowly taste it, taking as long as you can.
- Talk about the experience afterwards.
- Share each other's dimensions of what was noticed.

A Positive Approach to Teaching about Food and Nutrition

Strategies for teaching about food and nutrition include the following:

- Keep the focus of food and nutrition lessons positive, rather than critical, negative or blaming.
- Keep the emphasis on the practical and relevant aspects of food rather than the theoretical aspects of nutrients.
- Avoid using the term 'junk food' as it creates blame and guilt.
- Avoid focusing on sugar and unhealthy fats and keep the focus on the positive benefits of healthy foods.
- Encourage children to savour and enjoy what they eat.
- Explore many different types fruit and vegetables as a fun way to encourage healthy eating.
- Emphasise the key messages of variety, balance and moderation rather than 'good' and 'bad' foods.
- Be a sensible role model and do not make negative remarks about your own weight, diet or poor eating habits.
- Be seen choosing and enjoying healthy options.
- Encourage children to become involved in the preparation and enjoyment of healthy foods and snacks.
- Keep the focus on what children can enjoy rather than what they should avoid.
- Encourage children to enjoy cooking.

(Adapted from O'Dea, 2007)

Screen Time

An important aspect of the programme is challenging children to find something that is more fun to do than watching TV. Although children are watching less television, this does not mean that children have become more active as they are compensating by using computers to surf the Internet or play video games. Marion Nestle (2007) suggests that these sedentary visual activities amount to an average of 38 hours per week for the average child aged between two and 18 years of age. Recent studies suggest that watching TV and playing video games are the main contributors to a sedentary lifestyle leading to many hours each day of inactivity, time that could be used for engaging in moderate and vigorous physical activities. Television advertising leads to the consumption of food that is low in nutritional value. Encouraging pupils to limit the amount of television they watch frees up time for what positive psychologists call 'flow' activities such as art, music, riding bikes, dancing, drawing and reading.

Flow

Positive psychologist Mihaly Csikszentmihalyi (1990) describes flow as the mental state achieved when individuals are fully engaged in what they are doing. It is a feeling of energised focus, full of involvement and success in the process of the activity that is being undertaken. Flow can be experienced in any area of life where we are fully and completely involved, doing something for its own sake because we want to and because we are keen to take our skills to the next level. Flow provides us with the energy and commitment to do something with grit and persistence. It is a positive and practical outcome of self-motivated learning. Children who experience flow gain satisfaction from learning and are more likely to engage in future activities, which lead to flow. Electronic games can interfere with flow as they usually provide rewards at regular intervals. These rewards are often the appeal of the game. Children play to be rewarded rather than enjoying the process of play itself.

The Hard Business of Persuasion

Persuading children to make nutritious food choices and be physically active takes time. Having a trusted adult to encourage children to try something new and persist until they do, is absolutely crucial. This was clearly illustrated in Jamie Oliver's television series in 2005. Oliver went into a South London secondary school, Kidbrooke, with the aim of improving the quality of the lunches on offer. When one student at Kidbrooke, initially a new food refuser, was asked by Oliver why he had started eating the new and healthy meals, his answer was simple, it was 'Nora', the school's catering manager, or head dinner lady. Parent involvement in the programme will also help to boost its effectiveness. Encouraging parents and family members to become involved in activities at home that complement the key messages of the programme, increase the probability that the dietary and lifestyle changes that pupils make, will become a regular part of family and daily life, and therefore, help to safeguard our children's future health.

What is Health?

The World Health Organisation (1948) defines health as 'a state of complete physical, mental and social wellbeing and not merely the absence of disease or infirmity'.

Physical Health

Physical health often dominates our perception of overall health. The idea that healthy means 'not being sick' is a common viewpoint, but one that is very limited. Physical health encompasses immunity, physical growth, maintenance, and recovery from injury, overall function of the senses, susceptibility to disease and disorders, body functioning, stress management and recuperative ability. It also means having a healthy body weight and maintaining normal growth in childhood and adolescence.

Mental Health

Psychological or mental health includes a person's mental state, their mental functioning, and sense of psychological wellbeing. Children have sound mental health when they feel loved, respected, are safe and secure, and have a responsible adult taking care of them.

Psychosocial health in children is also characterised by a sense of self-worth, self-esteem, self-satisfaction and optimism about their place in the world and their future. Mental health also refers to a sense of resilience where children can develop the ability to learn from their mistakes and failure, and are able to bounce back and grow from the experience.

Social Health

Social health is crucial as children need to feel connected to others in order to flourish. Healthy relationships can help to mitigate the effects of stress and anxiety. A strong and stable social structure and being able to open up and talk to others about a variety of issues is essential for wellbeing. Feeling accepted and actively involved in cultural activities is also an important aspect of social health.

Emotional Health

Emotional health refers to a child's ability to identify and express their emotions when appropriate and have their emotional needs met. This means controlling the expression of emotions when it is appropriate to do so in an appropriate manner. Feelings of self-esteem, self-confidence, self-efficacy, trust, love and many other emotional reactions and responses are all part of a child's emotional health.

Spiritual Health

Spiritual health refers to a child's sense of belonging in the world. A child who is spiritually healthy feels that they have a place in the world, that life is important and valuable with meaning and purpose, and that their destiny will also be meaningful and fruitful.

Body Image

Health also includes having a positive body image. Jenny O'Dea (2007) explains that body image is the mental picture we have of our bodies and how we feel about our physical selves. It is a concept or scheme that includes feelings and perceptions such as awareness of the body, body boundaries, attention to parts of the body as well as to the whole, position in space and gender related perceptions.

Body image includes an individual's perception and judgement of the size, shape, weight and any other aspect of the body that relates to appearance. Body image is an important aspect of health for children.

Body image is multidimensional. It includes the way we view ourselves as well as the way that we believe others view us. Body image is not static. It changes in response to changing feedback from the environment.

How Body Image Develops

Body image develops based on interactions with the people and the world around us. Newborn infants view themselves as an extension of the mother. They do not make a distinction between their bodies and the world. They trust their mothers to take care of their needs, and mothers earn this trust by consistently responding to their infant's needs in a nurturing way.

As they develop, infants begin to sense that there is a boundary between their bodies and the rest of the world. They begin to be able to tell the difference between their bodies and other objects, and that their bodies are separate from the bodies of other people. At this stage, they become preoccupied with touching and tasting as they explore this new world.

Gradually, the boundary between the self and others becomes more distinct. With a higher level of self-awareness, children get a sense of their independence. Toddlers are eager to explore this new state of self-awareness. They often use the word 'no' to assert their newly discovered autonomy.

Parents and other caregivers can encourage toddlers' newfound sense of separateness by encouraging them to do things for themselves.

Toddlers tend to be curious about everything and are constantly on the move. They need clear limits for acceptable behaviour because they have no judgement, little self-control and immense energy.

Body image becomes more refined as children learn to enjoy using their bodies in recreational activities. Children are eager to climb structures, ride tricycles, run races and play catch. Adults often feel some conflict between fostering independence and protecting children from possible harm. At this stage, adults must set limits, while recognising that children need to develop physical skills. As children grow and develop, they are subject to influences beyond the primary caregivers in their lives. These social influences on body image continue throughout life. In the UK, the media is one of the most pervasive social influences. Hutchins and Calland (2011) write that our children's world is saturated with media images and within each image there is an implicit message about ideals, values and expectations. From social networking sites to mobile phones, iPlayers and computer games, children are bombarded with images of flawless, beautiful women and muscular, toned men. A study by Field et al. (2005) suggests that frequent exposure to these media messages is linked to low self-esteem, stress, insecurity and negative feelings in girls and young women.

Mass media, in cooperation with business, sells the 'perfect' body to us on a regular basis. Drink this beverage, eat this cereal, buy this piece of exercise equipment and you too can have the ideal body. We spend billions each year on weight control products and services to help us achieve the perfect body. The media promotes unrealistic expectations about our ability to attain this ideal. Many young people come to believe that they can have a certain body size and shape if they just buy or do the right things. This ignores the basic reality that human beings come in a wide variety of sizes and shapes, and fails to recognise that diversity is a positive characteristic of human beings. It perpetuates a society that ostracises and stigmatises people who deviate too greatly from the perceived ideal. Children come to believe that overweight children and adults have made the wrong decision or have no will power and thus deserve to be treated as outcasts or inferior beings. Research by Bryan (2003) shows that young children link being fat with being unintelligent, doing less well at school, being lazy, smelly and less liked by peers.

Reflections on Body Image (Swinson, 2012), a report published by the All Party Parliamentary Group on Body Image, found that children and young people are particularly vulnerable to social and cultural pressures to conform to unrealistic beauty ideals. The report suggests that a high proportion of children and young people have negative body images. Evidence submitted to the inquiry suggested that from about the age of five, children begin to recognise that they are different from other people and understand that they may be judged because of this. In particular, the inquiry found that children and young people are particularly vulnerable to social and cultural pressures to conform to unrealistic beauty ideals, and those who experience body dissatisfaction are likely to pursue the perfect body ideal in a variety of unhealthy ways, such as by dieting, excessive exercise and in extreme cases by vomiting and starvation. Research conducted in the UK and internationally, and submitted to the Inquiry reported that:

- between one third and half of young girls fear becoming fat and engage in dieting or binge eating

- one in four, seven year old girls have tried to lose weight at least once

- one third of young boys aged 8 to 12 are dieting to lose weight.

The report identified a clear need to equip young people with the tools to handle these pressures and ensure that they have the emotional resilience needed to withstand pressures and feel positive about themselves and their bodies.

Warning Signs

Warning signs that a child has developed a poor body image may include:

- a reluctance to take part in activities that involve undressing with others, such as swimming or PE

- withdrawing from social activities

- being unwilling to have a go at something new.

Parents should also be concerned if their child continually talks about themselves and their looks in a critical or negative way.

Self-Esteem

Self-esteem and body image are inextricably linked. Coopersmith (1967), in his classic work on self-esteem, defines it as the judgement we make about the worth of ourselves. Individuals with healthy levels of self-esteem are fundamentally satisfied with themselves while at the same time able to identify weaker characteristics that they may need to work on. Healthy self-esteem involves a realistic appraisal of the self's characteristics and competencies together with an attitude of self-acceptance, self-respect and self-worth.

Body image encompasses what we think of our physical bodies, while self-esteem includes our feelings about our own worth as individuals. Body image and self-esteem together create our self-concept, which is the fabric of how we feel about ourselves, making it difficult to separate the two. A child's self-concept starts to be constructed from a very early age and continues to develop throughout childhood. Encouraging a positive self-concept in a variety of domains is the key to building overall self-esteem in children and lowering the importance of physical appearance. Individuals with healthy self-esteem usually feel positive about their appearance, while people with low self-esteem are frequently dissatisfied with how they look. To reject the appearance or capabilities of our body is to reject an integral component of ourselves. Body weight and particularly overweight is recognised to be a reliable predictor of lower self-esteem. Studies of the relationship between self-esteem and body weight in children aged below 12 years of age have found an inverse relationship between self-esteem and measures of body weight. Lucy Cavendish (2011) writing about her overweight nine year old son suggests that:

> In a society that values thinness, Leonard is carrying around a terrible burden. It's one I try to keep from him. I try to gloss over it, tell him it's fine to be who he is (which it is because he is lovely). Like every overweight child though, he knows he is too big. Sometimes he gets unhappy about it. Sometimes he feels embarrassed. When he is feeling very low, he calls himself 'Lennie, the Lump' and it makes me want to cry.

Building self-esteem is generally recognised as being a logical approach to the prevention of body image and eating problems. Several decades ago, Bayer (1984) suggested the following advice for parents, educators and health professionals working with children and young people:

> Help young people feel good about themselves and accept themselves... avoid driving children to excel beyond their capabilities in academic or other endeavours and provide them with an appropriate but not unlimited degree of autonomy, choice, responsibility and self-accountability for their actions.

A healthy level of self-esteem is now recognised to be one of the most important protective factors in the development of resilience, as it contributes to positive social behaviours and provides a buffer against the impact of negative influences. An extensive study by Mann et al. (2004) suggests that poor self-esteem can play a critical role in the development of depression, anorexia nervosa, bulimia nervosa, other eating disorders, anxiety, violence, substance abuse, high risk behaviours and suicide. On the other hand, healthy self-esteem is protective against these problems and contributes to their prevention as well as the promotion of positive outcomes such as academic achievement, competence in a variety of domains, self-satisfaction, life satisfaction, resilience and coping ability.

Ways to Increase Children's Self-Esteem

- Positive psychologists emphasise what they call the 'power of salutation', that is, calling individuals by their name. Using the pupil's name helps them to understand that they are unique and valued individuals.

- Smile and let your students know that you enjoy their company.

- Treat your pupils with respect even when they are disrespectful to you or others.

- Enable pupils to identify and celebrate their unique strengths and talents.

- Notice when your pupils do something right rather than only noticing when they do something wrong.

- Praise and congratulate positive behaviours.

- Reward a pupil's positive attitude and effort, for example, 'I noticed how hard you worked on that task. Well done'.

- Do not give up on difficult pupils as they are the ones who need your support and reassurance the most.

- Establish firm but reasonable expectations for all pupils.

- Build up pupils' sense of efficacy and sense of mastery by enabling them to achieve rather than fail.

- Expect pupils to succeed and let them know that you believe in them.

- Never criticise a pupil in front of others.

(Adapted from O'Dea, 2007)

The Necessary Conditions for Self-Esteem

Reynold Bean (1992) identified four conditions that are necessary to maintain a healthy level of self-esteem:

1. A sense of connectedness.

2. A sense of uniqueness.

3. A sense of power.

4. A sense of role-models.

These four conditions refer to feelings that children have about themselves and the world around them. Children with healthy self-esteem experience all of these conditions in a variety of situations. Children with low self-esteem, on the other hand, have difficulty experiencing one or more of them.

A Sense of Connectedness

A strong and stable social network structure promotes overall health in individuals. Children with a high sense of being connected to others and belonging, are able to gain satisfaction from the people, places or things that they feel connected to. Positive interactions and relationships with others enable children to lead satisfying lives and buffer the effects of stress and anxiety. Feeling accepted and actively involved in cultural activities is an important aspect of health for many young people from cultural and ethnic backgrounds.

The Reflections on Body Image inquiry (Swinson, 2012) heard that experiences of discrimination and feelings of being different can undermine involvement in health education and social activities, for example, taking part in sport, participating in class discussions and socialising with others. If children are unhappy or uncomfortable with their body image, their sense of being securely connected to others is likely to suffer.

A Sense of Uniqueness

Children with a high sense of uniqueness, acknowledge and respect the qualities and characteristics they have that make them special and different. Acknowledgement from other people that these qualities and characteristics are important contribute to their sense of uniqueness. A strong sense of uniqueness allows children to express, respect and enjoy their own individuality.

Children whose body image does not fit the societal norm may feel unique in a negative way. Rather than being affirmed for what they are, they frequently feel judged for what they are not. If they feel that their individual qualities are not valuable or special, their sense of uniqueness suffers.

A Sense of Power

Children's sense of power is related to their belief in their own competence and in their ability to influence the circumstances of their lives. A strong sense of power enables children to take charge of important things in their lives, to make choices and to make desired changes.

Children who are considered to be overweight may be criticised by others for their behaviour around food and physical activity. This is especially the case if the adults who care for them attempt to limit their food intake. These children may begin to feel that they are incapable of controlling their own eating. Children who don't feel confidence in their bodies may not be able to direct the body's performance in physical activity. Such experiences are likely to have a negative effect on a child's sense of power.

A Sense of Role Models

Children need standards and values to help them make sense of the world. Role-models can be real or fictional people whose characteristics and actions we admire and seek to emulate. Philosophical models are the ideas, beliefs and values promoted by society, religion and families that guide our actions and choices. Finally, operational models are the automatic, almost subconscious responses and behaviours that develop as a result of constant, repetitive experiences. Social commentator, David Brooks (2011), writes that our character emerges gradually out of the mysterious interplay of a million little good influences. This model emphasises the power of community to shape character. Small habits and proper etiquette reinforce certain positive ways of seeing the world. Aristotle was right when he observed, 'We acquire virtues by first putting them into action'. Timothy Wilson (2011) of the University of Virginia puts it more scientifically:

> One of the most enduring lessons from social psychology is that behaviour change often precedes changes in attitude and feelings.

All these types of role models are reference points that guide behaviour and enable children to set their own goals, values, personal standards and ideals. In our weight-conscious society, children, especially overweight children, may have a difficult time finding positive role models. Similarly, children from a variety of cultural and ethnic backgrounds and those with disabilities may see few models to emulate in popular culture. This lack of role models emphasises children's differences in an unaffirming way. When we model respect for and acceptance of ourselves and others, regardless of body size or other physical attributes, we send a powerful message to our children that helps to build their self-esteem.

Being Sensitive to Body Image Issues

Children learn what is important to adults by listening to them and by watching them. When they hear adults expressing dissatisfaction with their bodies, they begin to believe that being an adult means being dissatisfied with your body. Similarly, when they hear adults being disparaging or critical about the bodies of others, they mimic this behaviour by teasing other children about their bodies. *The Reflections on Body Image* report (Swinson, 2012) commented:

> Children are affected by the people closest to them, so what their peer group says, what their parents say, what their teachers say, is going to be incredibly important.

It was suggested that parental concerns, such as throwaway comments about dieting or unhappiness with body size and appearance could be picked up and mimicked by children. The danger is that children do not possess the adult cognitive abilities and can absorb these 'throw away' remarks as facts. Kitty Hagenbach, a child and family therapist at the London parenting course specialist 'Babiesknow' comments:

> Children are really tuned into their parent's limbic brain and what you are thinking and feeling is picked up energetically in the atmosphere. A child knows what's going on even if you don't vocalise it. If there is any anxiety it can be very confusing for them.

> (Quoted in Cavendish, 29.10.11)

American clinical psychologist Dr Terese Weinstein Katz, the woman behind online resources www.eatsanely.com, offers this advice for absorbing children's anxiety:

> It's OK to say to your child, 'You know mummy has to watch it (her weight) because she's getting older, but you've got nothing to worry about'. That's much more understandable to a child than odd, anxious behaviour in their mother.

Be Aware of Your Own Body Image

Adults must ask themselves, what kind of role model am I for children with respect to body image? Teachers who are going to run the programme need to be aware of their influence on pupils as a powerful role models and may want to do the quiz at the end of this section.

Questions to Consider

Have I inadvertently promoted fear of fat in children by my attitude, words and actions?

Questions include:

- Am I dissatisfied with my body size and shape?
- Do I talk about my unhappiness with my body?
- Whom do I talk to, and who might overhear what I have to say?
- Am I always on a diet or about to go on one?
- Who knows when I am on a diet and how do they know?
- Do I express guilt when I eat certain foods?
- Do I refuse to eat certain foods while commenting that I am dieting to lose weight?
- Do I make negative comments about other people's sizes and shapes?
- Do I feel superior to them because I think my body is fitter than theirs?
- Am I prejudiced against overweight children and adults?
- Do I avoid making friends with overweight people?
- Am I embarrassed to be seen in public with overweight people?
- As a teacher, do I tend to pay less attention to overweight children in my classroom?

- Have I ever been surprised when an overweight child whom I thought was not very bright got a high score on a standardised test?

- Has a parent ever complained that I was treating an overweight child unfairly in some way?

(Adapted from Bacon, 2008)

Although these questions have no definitive answers, exploring one's responses to them can lead to personal resolutions for change. Actions to take may include the following:

- Developing a philosophy that it is not fair to judge others on the basis of their body size, shape, colour or other physical attributes.

- Recognising that the pursuit of thinness reflects a superficial value system and put a stop to self-criticism over failure to achieve the ideal body.

- Purchasing items from companies that make realistic claims in advertising or on labels.

- Pointing out unrealistic claims to children and helping them to understand that the purpose of advertising is to sell products.

We also need to be sensitive to body image issues other than weight, including height and physical abilities. As we strive to foster healthy body images in children, we should be consistent in promoting the following concepts:

- Individuals come in a variety of sizes and shapes and have different physical characteristics and abilities. This diversity should be accepted, respected and valued.

- We respect the bodies of others even when they are quite different from our own bodies.

- Everyone's body is a good body.

Fat Prejudice

As the UK becomes an increasingly multicultural society, more and more attention is given to issues of cultural and ethnic diversity and combating discrimination and prejudice. The importance of teaching children to accept, respect and value differences is now fully embedded in the policy and practice of schools and other settings. Body size, however, is one area in which diversity has not yet received widespread acceptance. Prejudice and discrimination against overweight or fat individuals may be one of the last acceptable prejudices. This could be linked to the reported widespread under-recognition by parents, teachers and health professionals of the prevalence and seriousness of obesity in children and adolescents reported by Parry (2008) and Baur (2005).

Children's Literature

Evidence of fat prejudice can be found in children's literature. Preceded by Frank Richards' (1950) Billy Bunter and William Golding's (1954) character Piggy, in Lord of the Flies, J.K. Rowling's immensely popular Harry Potter stories are an example of the disrespect that overweight children receive. She writes that Harry's heroic qualities shame those of his cousin Dudley, a stupid, cowardly bully, pampered by his parents and constantly tormenting Harry. But Dudley's worst attribute, which follows him from early childhood to adolescence, is his fatness. In several episodes that clearly target the humour created by such stereotypes but ignore the hurt that they may cause to fat children as readers, Dudley's obese eating behaviour attracts ridicule and punishment. Throughout the series the characterisation of a fat child never wavers.

J. K. Rowling's (2000) fourth book in the Harry Potter series, Goblet of Fire, continues to emphasise Dudley's fatness. At this point the boys are in early adolescence and Harry comments, 'Dudley's diet isn't going too well because he is always smuggling doughnuts into his room'. His parents attempt to replace Dudley's favourite foods, fizzy drinks, cakes, chocolate bars and burgers with fruit and vegetables. In the end, however, 'Dudley had finally achieved what he's been threatening to do since the age of three and become wider than he is tall'.

Sharron Dalton (2004) notes that none of the extensive commentary on the Harry Potter books, though sometimes critical of their religious implications, mentions the author's portrayal of Dudley and the obvious fat discrimination that it represents.

Dalton writes:

> Rowling is clearly determined to mine the joke of Dudley's body size for all its worth. But her humour is not funny. No child makes such a determination. In reality, the culprits are not children of any size or persuasion, but rather ignorance and insensitivity from an uncaring and uninformed society.

Dalton questions how many millions of readers respond to this characterisation of Dudley's agony as Harry does, with a mix of disgust, laughter and ridicule? In a culture suffering from an increase of obesity and fat phobia, how many other readers will look in the mirror and see an image of Dudley? Dalton suggests that the Harry Potter books are just one example of prejudice that routinely associates fatness with rude, offensive behaviour by ugly brats who are justly punished precisely because of their food habits. Insidious social discrimination appears as humour, but nevertheless carries a lethal message that making fun of fat children, and in extreme cases, physically bullying and hurting them, is acceptable because they deserve it. This portrayal of Dudley worsens the problem of childhood obesity by creating stereotypes and undermining the self-esteem of those overweight children who most need attention and assistance, as they work hard to modify both their eating and physical inactivity.

Tackling fat discrimination is an important part of helping overweight children achieve and maintain a healthy weight, because society's intolerance towards fat bodies can exacerbate the problem thus making fat children even fatter. Dr Linda Bacon (2008), associate nutritionist at the University of California and founder of the 'Health At Every Size' movement (www.haesbook.com) writes:

> With all these health experts and professionals telling us to lose weight it just makes people bigger. Fat or thin, we are scared of fat and feel bad about it and when people feel bad about themselves they make bad choices and eat more.

Dalton (2004) observes that parents never emerge as heroes in the novels of children who struggle in the face of fat discrimination. They are not up to the task of positively reinforcing their children or giving them the unconditional love that they clearly need. Dalton suggests that the stories can, however, provide a useful source of dos and don'ts for all those who are working to combat discrimination against overweight children. Talking about children's fiction that confronts fatness at home or in the classroom can air tensions and resolve conflicts. Dalton urges parents and teachers not to miss this opportunity for learning. Unlike restrictive dieting for children which does not establish healthy lifelong patterns, reading and talking about body size and feelings towards others who tease or bully will enable children to deal with their own unique body size and shape. A selection of children's literature providing insight into childhood obesity can be found at the end of Part Four.

There is no doubt, however, that fighting fat discrimination is challenging because in enabling children to form their own values, parents struggle with contradictory social messages about beauty versus social tolerance. In our culture, thinness has become synonymous with beauty and fatness with ugliness, and from an early age children learn that western culture judges attractiveness and social acceptability using body shape and size as an important criteria. The ideals of slimness for both males and females are learned from early childhood and the stereotypical slim female and muscular male are well-entrenched in young people who seek the success, admiration, social approval and attractiveness that attaining these ideals offers. It is not surprising that fear of fat has become endemic among both adults and children in our society.

A recent online poll of 1,500 children aged between seven and 18, carried out by Onepoll and Youngpoll quoted in *The Times* (29.10.2011) revealed that almost one quarter of children under ten consider themselves overweight. 26 per cent of the children had skipped a meal in the hope of losing weight, while nearly a quarter of them had already been on a diet in the past year. Two thirds of children aged seven to ten admitted to weighing themselves and more than half of all the girls said that they wanted to be a size ten or smaller when they grew up. By the time they are six years old, most children think that being fat is 'bad'. When they are asked to describe overweight children, studies suggest that six years olds will use negative adjectives such as 'lazy', 'sloppy', 'dirty' and 'stupid'.

The desire to become slimmer and the presence of weight-losing behaviours have been reported in children as young as seven years. Studies show that body image and eating disturbances among girls increase with age and in particular there is dissatisfaction with upper thighs, buttocks and stomach measurements. Although the pressures are sometimes less obvious for boys, they nevertheless still exist. Pursuing these body image ideals can be very unhealthy for children and young people as they are likely to damage their physical, psychological and social health in their quest for bodily perfection.

Media Literacy

While overweight children may hear messages such as 'you must diet' and 'you must exercise' there are many other strong influences in their daily lives that shape the choices that they make from television advertisements and billboards, to what's in the vending machine or what toy comes with a meal at a fast food restaurant. Marion Nestle (2007) lists the marketing methods that target children outside of school as follows:

- television advertising
- internet advertising
- magazine advertising
- internet interactive computer games
- toys, clothing, telephone cards and other items with logos
- celebrity endorsement of products
- product placement in films

- supermarket positioning of items
- fast food chain toys and gifts, prizes

Parents can encourage children, through their own example, to be aware of the relentless media pressures to look a certain way, and help them to foster a questioning and challenging approach to society's rigid ideals of thinness and the media images that they are presented with.

The term 'media literacy' refers to an individual's ability to decipher media messages and see through the hype. Media literacy enables children and young people to become aware of the media's influence in their lives, and to understand how it operates to create messages and 'sell' ideas and products. Media literacy also teaches children how media messages can be educational and helpful as well as inaccurate and untruthful, promoting unhealthy attitudes and behaviours. Children are taught how to take these messages apart to show how they are made and that they are not necessarily true.

The Emotional Consequences of Being Overweight

The emotional consequences of being overweight are far beyond what most families realise. Overweight children are likely to feel bad about themselves because society feels bad about them and despises fat. Sylvia Rimm (2004) describes the trauma that overweight children frequently experience when she writes:

> Children and adults alike don't seem to feel guilty when making offensive comments, almost as if they believe that they have a right to punish children who are overweight. Adults often mistakenly believe that challenging or even sarcastic comments will encourage children to lose weight, however, the psychological impact of this prejudice generally provokes children to eat even more and exercise less.

It is important for teachers to understand what perpetuates the vicious cycle of overweight that typically begins between the ages of four to seven years.

Nature and Nurture

The Role of Heredity

Both weight and height are the result of the interaction of genetics and the environment.

A discussion with children about heredity and the difference between things we can change and things we can't change can be especially helpful for children who have concerns about body size. Adults can encourage children to accept body characteristics that can't be changed by modelling such acceptance of their own bodies. Adults can also model making healthy choices to increase their fitness.

Studies by Le Grange and Lock (2011) suggest that parental overweight is the single most important predictor of weight problems in children under the age of six years. Heredity also comes into play, but it is not the dominant source of the condition. Scientists have discovered the so-called obesity gene. This gene produces leptin, a hormone that affects how the body processes fat and appears to regulate how much energy the body expends to sustain itself. Other genes are involved in the process too, regulating such things as metabolism, appetite and fat storage. Recent research studies suggest that genes are responsible for an estimated 30-50 per cent of how an individual's body regulates weight. However, although genetic makeup may predispose the condition, it is the child's environment that causes it.

Environmental Influences

Environmental influences refer to the family's eating and activity habits. Obese parents may have food and activity habits that foster their obesity. Children of obese parents may acquire such habits from their parents. If genetics determine 30-50 per cent of weight regulation, that means a significant 50-70 per cent is attributed to environment, something that it is possible to control. The effect of genetics has not changed in the past three decades or so as human genes take thousands of years to change. The rapid increase in the number of overweight children must therefore be due to the environment. The family home in general has an enormous influence on the child's health and wellbeing. Environmental components include:

- types of food, how much and how often a child eats.
- the family's attitude towards food.
- the family's eating habits.
- the types of activities the family engage in such as sports, watching television, computer games, family outings, dancing, playing cards.
- the emotional culture in the home.

If a child has one or two obese parents or the oldest sibling is overweight the chances of the younger child becoming overweight goes up. With each additional member of the family who is overweight, the risk increases. On the other hand, children who have two lean parents and no overweight siblings have a much lower risk of becoming overweight.

When one child in the family is obese the results can be devastating. As Cavendish (2011) identifies:

> The most disconcerting thing is that we are not a fat family. Often when you see a fat child, the mother, father and the siblings are also large, generally due to poor nutrition and a dependence on takeaway food and sugary snacks. But we are not that family. Everyone else in my family is normal sized and has the appropriate BMI. Leonard is the only one whose waistbands don't fit. We all eat the same food, do the same amount of exercise, but Leonard is a round roly-poly pudding and the rest of us are not.

The bottom line is that although genes contribute to weight problems, the family environment has the greatest impact upon a child's weight. The flip side of this fact is that the family environment also has the greatest impact on the child's ability to lose weight, keep it off and build a healthy life style.

The Emotions of Food and Exercise

It is important to recognise when seeking to address the difficulties associated with food, faced by overweight children, that food in our society is about much more than nutrition.

Food is Love

Food in our society is primarily about love. When a newborn baby cries, one of the first comforts that we provide is food and later we think that a miserable toddler is probably a hungry child and guess that tears communicate hunger. Children who have just been fed usually smile or sleep peacefully. If food is about love then the withdrawal of food is the withdrawal of love, care and nurturing.

Food is Health

Food is also health, and all cultures tend to associate chubby babies with health and contentment. They prove that we are successful parents. 'Eat, my child, and grow healthy and strong' translates into any language and through all cultures and if fat babies prove that we are successful parents, how can we risk serving our children less food?

Food is Celebration

As a society we are conditioned to celebrating with food, and the more special the occasion the more likely the food will be plentiful, fattening and unhealthy. Family and friends relationships at every stage are celebrated by food. Because we are so conditioned to celebrating birthdays, holidays, graduations, weddings with delicious food it seems inappropriate and uncomfortable to celebrate with less food and with non-fattening foods. Dara-Lynn Weiss (2012) describing her painful struggle to control the weight of Bea, her seven year old daughter writes:

> School is a particular challenge… who is protecting the obese kids when the 350-calorie cupcakes are handed out to the entire class on every kid's birthday? Who's informing parents of the sugary treats distributed freely at Halloween? And ice cream the day before the spring break? And pizza in honour of the class's good behaviour? In a situation where a single Hershey's Miniature needs to be accounted for, this freewheeling distribution of high-calorie snacks is a menace to my child's health.

Food is Basic

Food is a necessity and we can't live without it. Too much unhealthy and delicious food will always be there to tempt us. Food pleases our palates and we enjoy its taste. Even if we aren't celebrating or proclaiming our love or friendship, we enjoy eating.

Food is Power

Children quickly learn that food provides them with power. To eat or not to eat can affect how adults relate to each other or how they treat their children at mealtimes or snack time. Some children direct the dinner table with their refusal to eat anything or their insistence on eating too much or too little. Dara Lynn Weiss (2012) writes about putting her seven year old daughter Bea on a diet:

> Though I knew the process would be emotional and difficult, I hadn't anticipated the degree to which I would be treated like a pariah by the people around me. 'You're making her crazy' was a popular observation. 'You should let her eat what she wants, she's still a little kid' some argued. 'She's still growing' some argued. 'I'd never put my kid on a diet' many parents pronounced. There was dissent within my own family.

Food Can Become a Problem

When the chubbiness of infancy doesn't disappear and we notice a child's plumpness we try not to talk about it and deny there's a weight problem until a doctor's check up confirms that there is a problem. Cavendish (2011) describes her experience of having a child who is overweight:

> How can I explain the difficulties, the pain of having a child who is overweight? I spend night after night, day after day wondering why Leonard is so much bigger than the rest of us. I lie awake at night wondering what to do about it. I have tried just about everything, endless courses, trips to the doctor, clinics at my local hospital and yet... Leonard just gets bigger and bigger and I'm not actually sure why. My antennae are always up. I have to bite my tongue not to tell him, 'That's enough', 'No seconds for you'. I monitor what he eats constantly.

Once it is confirmed that a child is overweight we are forced to change role from giving food to withdrawing or limiting it. Children manipulate adults even more as their overweight causes them to feel powerless in a peer society that is destructive and prejudiced against overweight children. It would appear that increasingly overweight and being 'fat' is becoming a class issue. According to figures from the National Obesity Observatory (NOO, 2007), an organisation established to provide authoritative data on the obesity epidemic, females who have careers in fields such medicine, the law or business are the only social group to lose weight in the past 15 years. As Cavendish (2011) comments, society has the perception that it is the lower socioeconomic groups who are breeding a new generation of children who are too fat and writes:

> Let's face it, nobody wants their child to look like a chav. Sometimes I find it embarrassing my son is obese. I know I shouldn't. I know it's not personal, but that's how it feels. I live in a resolutely middle-class area. Children in this part of the country aren't fat. It is almost a criminal act to be fat where I live... As soon as Leonard puts anything fattening into the shopping trolley, crumpets, for example, I whip them out with a flourish, 'Oh we don't need them' I'll say as if to show the other shoppers that it's not my fault he is overweight.

Weiss (2012) writes that:

> In 2011 a Kelton Research survey revealed that parents find the single most uncomfortable topic to discuss with their kids is not sex, not drugs, but weight. The reasons for this are obvious: In a culture rife with eating disorders and ominous warnings of how tenuous kids' self-esteem is, especially among girls, telling a seven year old that she has to lose weight is not only uncomfortable it is almost unimaginable. So parents often do what I have done, they ignore the problem. What's more I felt acutely ill-prepared to deal with this particular challenge.

The Emotions of Exercise

Sharron Dalton (2004) writes that discrimination against overweight children often pushes them to eat more and exercise less.

As we think about how to encourage children to develop healthy eating habits we also have to consider how to encourage them to become more active. Exercise, like food, however, can also be fraught with emotions. Healthy toddlers tend to be curious about everything and are constantly on the move. They gradually learn to enjoy using their bodies in a range of recreational activities. Children are eager to climb structures, ride bicycles, run races and play team games. In what Tim Gill (2007) calls our 'risk averse society' adults often feel some conflict between fostering children's independence and at the same time protecting them from possible harm. Overweight children present a different challenge, as adults notice that they avoid exercise and instead prefer to immerse themselves in lethargic inactivity. They prefer to sit, watch TV, play computer games, draw, read and do puzzles. When they are encouraged to join in physical activity, they typically protest, make excuses and argue. Dalton (2004) observes that getting teased about being overweight frequently occurs during times when children are engaging in physical activity. Children who can't run fast or whose heavy thighs are on display draw the unwanted attention of their peers.

The Vicious Cycle

Although overweight children may get labelled 'lazy' it is, in fact, frequently their size that limits their active involvement in the playground and sports hall. Their extra weight can result in reduced endurance and leg pain from stressed joints. Physical activity becomes increasingly demanding. Less ability to move, combined with reduced skill and confidence, means that overweight children retreat indoors, are likely to take comfort in snacking in front of the TV set and conclude that exercise is not for them. This lack of physical activity is likely to result in continued weight gain. Practitioners working with overweight children are usually all too aware of the vicious circle that ensues. Overweight children are caught at every turn of the wheel. Teasing and even bullying in the lunch hall can lead to:

- unhealthy eating habits
- unhealthy food behaviours
- hiding food
- emotional eating
- binge eating.

As practitioners we feel sorry for overweight children as they escape back to television, books, art or computers. Overall, they avoid physical activity and although we know that they should stay active part of us, suggests Dalton (2004), may be feels relieved from the embarrassment of their awkward participation.

Discrimination against overweight children by other children and adults often pushes them to eat more and exercise less. Bacon (2008) writes of 'emotional eating':

> Many of us come to view food as blanket for our emotions, numbing them as we turn to food to provide the love and comfort we crave. Food is reward, friend, love and support. We eat not because we are hungry but because we're sad, guilty, bored, frustrated, lonely or angry. In doing so, we're ignoring those internal hard-wired hunger and fullness signals. And because there's no way that food can really address our emotions, we eat and eat and eat but never feel satisfied.

It is also essential that overweight children feel encouraged not embarrassed during physical activity. We readily praise children who excel at sports, yet those on the sidelines are often the ones who most need our support and encouragement. Fighting fat discrimination may improve the quality of life for fat children by improving their psychological wellbeing and it also addresses their risk of physical disease because an improvement in psychological wellbeing leads to improvement of the other. Children who are comfortable in their relationships with others in the classroom and in the playground and who participate freely in sports and other opportunities for achievement usually find a balance in eating and sedentary activity.

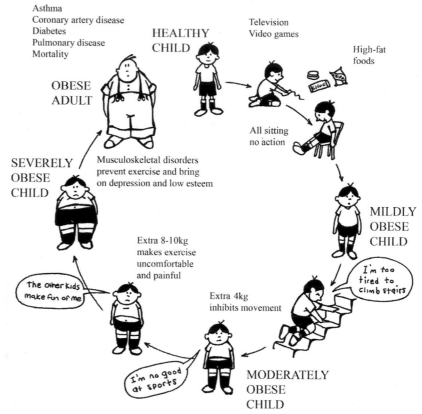

Fat discrimination feeds the cycle of overeating, reduced physical activity and lower self-esteem.

Adapted from The Vicious Cycle of Childhood Obesity (Committed to Kids, 2002). www. committed-to-kids.com

Addressing Fat Discrimination

Despite the growing problem of fat discrimination against children and young people there are very few academic studies that address this. Sondra Solovay's (2000) *Tipping the Scales of Justice* explores how fat discrimination is entirely predictable and the resulting devastation is foreseeable. These experiences result in lower self-esteem, alienation and denial of the benefits of activity while unnecessarily curtailing children's future opportunities. Protecting every fat child from all harassment is impossible, but some basic improvements have to be made. Specifically, parents and the public need to be educated and to educate themselves about fat prejudice in order to alleviate some of the intense, cultural pressure put on children to lose weight no matter what the cost. It is unfair that children should be treated differently by their families, peers, caregivers and teachers just because they come in a 'larger package'. Improving the quality of life for fat children, emphasises Solovay, must become a priority for all people who are interested in a just society. Children who are concerned about their body size should be assured that they are lovable and capable just as they are. They need to understand that individuals come in small, medium and large sizes, and that their bodies will change as they grow. Children must be taught that their growing bodies need healthy food, exercise and sleep. When children learn to accept and respect the diversity of human appearance, they are better able to love their bodies for what they are and to choose to take care of them. When health rather than thinness is made the goal, everyone's body can attain its own ideal condition.

When a family struggles with parenting an overweight child, they often feel alone with their problem. The impact of being overweight on children's mental state should not be overlooked. It is important that practitioners understand that being overweight can have a devastating effect on a child's wellbeing. It can undermine a child's emotional health and have a negative impact upon the child's academic, social and emotional development. Lifestyle changes, however, will not be effective unless the emotional crisis that overweight children may be experiencing is dealt with.

Resilience

Resilience experts Robert Brooks and Sam Goldstein (2001) suggest that whatever we want for our children, be it happiness, friendship and connectedness, academic success, or satisfaction with their lives:

> Realisation of these goals requires that children have the inner strength to deal competently and successfully, day after day, with the challenges and demands that they encounter. They call that capacity to cope and feel competent, *resilience*.

If children in general need to develop resilience in order to deal effectively with stress and pressure, overweight children need it more in order to ensure that they can:

- cope with the everyday challenges that they face
- bounce back from disappointments
- take risks
- solve problems
- treat themselves with respect.

These skills and competencies, if learned early, can go a long way towards preventing the behaviours and series of events that lead to a child becoming overweight or obese.

Bubble Wrapped Children

Tim Gill (2007), one of the UK's leading writers and thinkers on childhood, argues that children's resilience and autonomy is being undermined by the growth of risk aversion that is intruding into many aspects of children's lives. Many adults increasingly view the world as a hostile place in which to raise children, and think that the solution is to create for them a risk free environment. This risk aversion restricts children's play, limits their freedom of movement, and constrains their exploration of the physical and social world.

Gill emphasises that choice, autonomy and freedom are essential for children's wellbeing and argues for a philosophy of resilience that will help counter risk aversion, and strike a better balance between protecting children from genuine threats and giving them rich, challenging opportunities from which they can learn.

Thanks to positive psychologists it is becoming increasingly recognised that the best way to support children is not by protecting them from challenges but by enabling them to develop resilience. Tal Ben-Shahar (2007) argues that the experience of overcoming difficulties, and successfully negotiating new challenges is vital to the development and maintenance of coping skills, and when challenged, children, like adults, will find meaning in their accomplishments and benefit from overcoming setbacks. Ben-Shahar goes as far as to say that struggles and challenges are actually good for us. Although as adults our immediate response is to want to make things easier for children, there are times when we have to curb this impulse and allow them the 'privilege of hardship'. Through discovering their psychological strength, children gradually learn how to take charge of their lives. This is because resilience:

- strengthens an individual
- enables us to have a go at new experiences
- allows us to accept challenges willingly
- helps us to cope with frustration and failure
- sustains us through hardship
- helps us work towards our goals and aspirations.

(Adapted from MacConville, 2012)

According to the renowned psychoanalyst Boris Cyrulnik (2009), who works with traumatised children internationally, resilience should not be confused with simply surviving or getting through, as some individuals can become trapped as victims, nursing their wounds and blocked from growth by anger and blame. Resilient individuals are able to transform their pain into something stronger.

Adults who have an understanding of resilience can cultivate a similar mindset and encourage resilient behaviours in their children. Key skills that are important for children to develop include:

- problem-solving
- breaking a task into smaller parts and mastering each item
- gaining the support of helpful others
- persisting in one's efforts.

Emotional Eating

If children learn self-nurturing and take care of their needs in a healthy way, such as playing a game with a friend when bored, setting limits for controlling urges for more food or TV, they are likely to avoid 'emotional eating'. Emotional eating has been defined as, '... eating in response to a range of negative emotions such as anxiety, depression, anger and loneliness to cope with negative effect' (Faith et al., 1997).

Boutelle and Tanofsky-Kraff (2011) write that emotional eating is a maladaptive or unhelpful coping strategy because it may provide short-term relief, but in the longer term it does not support the child. Children who are resilient and self-nurturing will find comfort and pleasure from sources other than food, such as having friends and being connected to others, engaging in physical activities and games. Parents can help build their child's resilience and healthy responses to stress by maximising their child's opportunities for:

- engaging in hobbies and interests
- building friendships
- making a contribution

• being aware of strengths and talents.

Cavendish (*The Times*, 2011) describing her guilt as a mother of nine year old Leonard who is an overweight child writes:

> His desire to fill himself up with food could also be his desire for more love/attention/ time from me. I try to find space for him and me to do activities together, just the two of us, each week. At the moment we are madly into trampolining.

Guidelines for Building Resilience

One barrier to developing resilience in children is that the adults themselves lack the characteristics that help build resilience in children. These include:

• the ability to be empathic
• being communicative
• being positive rather than negative
• being optimistic rather than pessimistic
• being realistic about their own strengths and weaknesses themselves.

The good news, suggests Robert Brooks and Sam Goldstein (2001), is that these abilities can be learned. In looking to reverse the childhood obesity epidemic the first step is to develop resilient children.

Strategies for Raising Resilient Children

1. Be Empathic

It is important that adults convey empathy as a way of fostering children's strengths, hopes and optimism. This means accepting children for who they are and helping them set realistic expectations and goals. Dan Goleman's (2006) concept of emotional intelligence can be construed as another name for empathy. Goleman names empathy as the fundamental 'people skill'.

Parents who are eager for their child's success may urge their overweight child to 'try harder'. Instead of holding the belief that a child must have a certain body size and shape in order to gain popularity with friends, or expect a child to excel in sports or school achievement, parents need to evaluate whether their expectations and goals are realistic and reasonable.

2. Focus on Strengths to Develop a Positive Self-Concept

Empathic parents put themselves inside the shoes of their children in order to appreciate their point of view. Doing this is easy when things are going well and children are responsive, but can be difficult to do when we are upset or disappointed with them. Adults who are empathic towards the challenge of obesity, look out for their child's strengths and identify them. Educational psychologist and writer Roffey (2011) explains that children develop a view of themselves that they have been given by adults since their early years. This may include 'lazy', 'nuisance', 'careless'. If you tell a boy how careless and clumsy he is, this is how he will see himself and have nothing to aim for. If you tell the same child how helpful he is, he will try to be helpful. This is not ignoring the problems, but focusing on what is going well and looking towards strengths. Working from a strengths perspective is more motivating than addressing entrenched deficits and problems. Studies by Barbara Frederickson (2009) confirm what common sense would suggest, that children become capable, productive and resilient when we identify and nurture their strengths rather than give attention to their deficits.

Dalton (2004) suggests that overweight children often have high levels of emotional intelligence, and are better at empathy than their parents because they have usually developed a keen sense of what it means to be different. They are able to display empathy towards other children who are also different. Cavendish (2011) describes her overweight son Leonard as:

> …a lovely, stoic sort of boy. He has the kindest heart I have ever known in a child… he is a very likeable boy and therefore popular boy. He is, thank goodness, not socially excluded.

3. Communicate Effectively and Listen Actively

By listening carefully to what children say, rather than telling them what they should be feeling, parents effectively communicate and develop resilience in children. It is important that children's fears and worries are taken seriously and that they feel heard. Parents who actively encourage opinions, discussions and expressions of individuality will help their children to feel valued and worthwhile.

4. Story Editing

Story editing is an approach that seeks to redirect an individual's interpretation of themselves and the world around them. It involves giving a child a different story or account of a situation in the hope that it will 'bump' them out of self-defeating thinking patterns and enable them to build up a view of themselves that is positive, solution focused and in line with their strengths. Adults often nag their children using the same script for years. Changing the script and instead of making negative comments, focusing on something that the child is doing successfully can show the child other possibilities. Reframing any issue can be hard and takes attention and practice.

5. Build 'Islands of Competence'

Enable children to experience success by identifying and reinforcing what Brooks and Goldstein (2001) call 'islands of competence'. These are the things that children are good at and enjoy. Building up a child's competences is a vital part of enabling that individual to become resilient. When children's self-esteem is at a low ebb and they feel hopeless, it's usually very difficult for them to hear anything positive about themselves. One solution is to engage the child in learning a new skill or something that the child has already mastered. 'Islands of competence' emphasise strengths rather than weaknesses and create opportunities for the child to flourish. Children should be encouraged to set goals and targets, and talk about their aims, hopes and ambitions.

6. Let Children Know that Mistakes are Experiences from which to Learn

Nobody intuitively views mistakes as opportunities for learning. Children typically experience mistakes as failures and may retreat from further challenges and feel inadequate. Encourage children to see mistakes as opportunities from which to learn.

7. Love Children in Ways that Make them Feel Special and Appreciated

Children need to develop a healthy self-esteem and feel good about themselves. It is this inner feeling of worth that helps insulate children from anxiety about their appearance and the need to conform to unrealistic ideals of physical attractiveness.

A basic ingredient for resilience is the presence of at least one adult who believes in the child's worth. This belief helps direct the child towards a productive and satisfying life. The late Dr Julius Segal (1988) referred to these individuals as 'charismatic adults' from whom a child 'gathers strength' and can therefore have a direct influence on the child's developing sense of self. For children, knowing that someone cares for them and is interested in their lives can improve their self-esteem and enhance their capacity to flourish.

Body Image Quiz

Have I inadvertently promoted fear of fat in children by my attitude, words and actions? You may wish to reflect on any relevant question.

Am I dissatisfied with my body size and shape?
Reflection:

Do I talk about my unhappiness with my body?
Reflection:

Whom do I talk to, and who might overhear what I have to say?
Reflection:

Am I always on a diet or about to go on one?
Reflection:

Who knows when I am on a diet and how do they know?
Reflection:

Do I express guilt when I eat certain foods?
Reflection:

Do I refuse to eat certain foods while commenting that I am dieting to lose weight?
Reflection:

Do I make negative comments about other people's sizes and shapes?
Reflection:

Body Image Quiz (Cont)

Do I feel superior to them because I think my body is fitter than theirs?
Reflection:

Am I prejudiced against overweight children and adults?
Reflection:

Do I avoid making friends with overweight people?
Reflection:

Am I embarrassed to be seen in public with overweight people?
Reflection:

As a teacher, do I tend to pay less attention to overweight children in my classroom?
Reflection:

Have I ever been surprised when an overweight child whom I thought was not very bright got a high score on a standardised test?
Reflection:

Has a parent ever complained that I was treating an overweight child unfairly in some way?
Reflection:

(Adapted from Bacon, 2008)

Part Two: Staff Preparation

PowerPoint Presentation

General Guidance on Delivering the Programme

Guidance on Practical Aspects of Delivering
the Programme

Working with Parents

PowerPoint Presentation

This section provides a PowerPoint presentation of 20 slides with additional notes and a range of activities to support the facilitator in delivering the presentation. The activity pages can be found after the last slide.

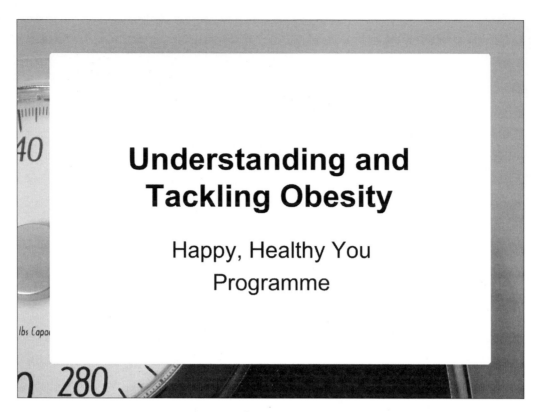

Understanding and Tackling Obesity

Happy, Healthy You

Programme

Facilitator Notes for Slide 1

The purpose of the presentation is to enable staff to understand the issues surrounding the current epidemic of obesity in children and young people, and how to tackle them. The presentation also introduces Happy, Healthy You, an intervention programme designed to proactively teach children positive living skills. This presentation provides practitioners with a guide to delivering the programme.

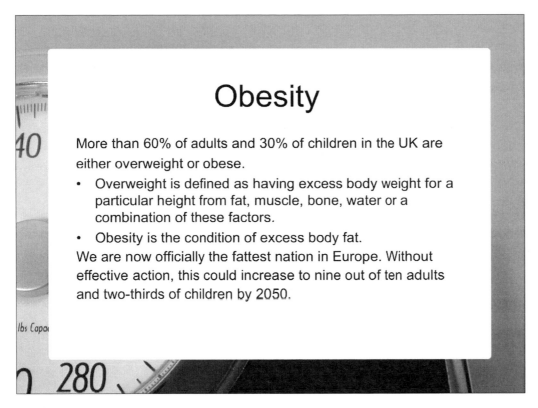

Obesity

More than 60% of adults and 30% of children in the UK are either overweight or obese.

- Overweight is defined as having excess body weight for a particular height from fat, muscle, bone, water or a combination of these factors.
- Obesity is the condition of excess body fat.

We are now officially the fattest nation in Europe. Without effective action, this could increase to nine out of ten adults and two-thirds of children by 2050.

Facilitator Notes for Slides 2 and 3

Obesity is the condition of increased body fat. It is the state of being seriously overweight, to a degree that affects your health.

Increasing obesity in childhood has been described as a 'time-bomb'. It already costs the NHS more than smoking does and if it continues to rise at the present rate, by 2023 there will be a 54% increase in Type 2 diabetes. Obesity is also widely recognised as being more difficult to deal with. The message to smokers is straightforward, 'stop smoking', but it is not possible to address obesity in such simple terms.

Activity Linked to Slides 2 and 3

Ask participants to comment on these facts and whether in their daily work with young people they are aware that an increasing number are either obese or overweight.

Obesity (Cont)

This increase in childhood obesity has received substantial media attention recently, partly due to the rapid increase in occurrence across the UK, as well as internationally. This rise began to occur in the UK in the mid 1980s, with a rapid increase occurring most noticeably over the following ten years. Current statistics suggest that the trend in obesity now appears to be flattening out. However, it will be important to continue to monitor the trends in future to confirm that this is a continuing pattern, rather than a plateau within a longer-term trend that is gradually increasing.

(ASO, 2011)

Slide 3

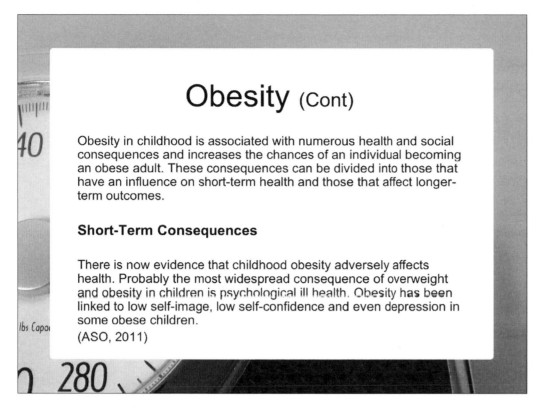

Obesity (Cont)

Obesity in childhood is associated with numerous health and social consequences and increases the chances of an individual becoming an obese adult. These consequences can be divided into those that have an influence on short-term health and those that affect longer-term outcomes.

Short-Term Consequences

There is now evidence that childhood obesity adversely affects health. Probably the most widespread consequence of overweight and obesity in children is psychological ill health. Obesity has been linked to low self-image, low self-confidence and even depression in some obese children.

(ASO, 2011)

Facilitator Notes for Slide 4

The social and psychological consequences for children who are overweight or obese can include stigmatisation, discrimination and prejudice. The 'Reflections on Body Image' Report published by the All Party Parliamentary Group on Body Image (Swinson, 2012) suggests that even young children are aware of the negative view held by society towards overweight and obese individuals and that this has a negative impact upon their developing sense of self and self-esteem. The extent to which obesity influences an obese child's self esteem varies from one child to another, although there are suggestions that obese adolescents may be more affected than younger children.

Activity Linked to Slide 4

Ask participants for their views on the link between low self-image, low self-confidence and even depression in obese and overweight children.

Take feedback.

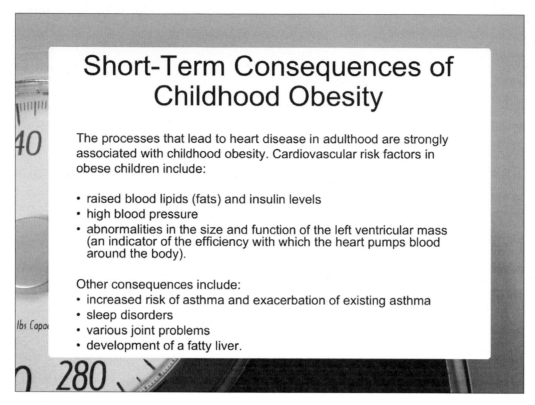

Short-Term Consequences of Childhood Obesity

The processes that lead to heart disease in adulthood are strongly associated with childhood obesity. Cardiovascular risk factors in obese children include:

- raised blood lipids (fats) and insulin levels
- high blood pressure
- abnormalities in the size and function of the left ventricular mass (an indicator of the efficiency with which the heart pumps blood around the body).

Other consequences include:
- increased risk of asthma and exacerbation of existing asthma
- sleep disorders
- various joint problems
- development of a fatty liver.

Facilitator Notes for Slides 5 and 6

The overall effect of all of these adverse consequences of childhood obesity is an increased risk of ill health and premature death in adult life. Both the short and longer-term consequences of childhood obesity are very serious for children's overall wellbeing and their physical health.

Activity Linked to Slides 5 and 6

Provide an opportunity for participants to comment on these facts about the health consequences of childhood obesity.

Longer-Term Consequences of Childhood Obesity

- A marked increase in the risk of ill health in adulthood that arises from obesity in childhood, independent of adult weight.
- Persistence of obesity from childhood and adolescence to adulthood. It is estimated that 70% of obese children and more than 85% of obese adolescents will become obese adults.
- For adolescents and young adults who are obese there is increased risk of lower educational attainment, social isolation and low income.

Slide 6

How Do We Know if a Child is Obese?

Just looking at a child is not enough to determine whether they are overweight or obese. Judgements made by just looking at the child or young person are often incorrect even when made by health professionals (Smith, 2008).

It is agreed that childhood overweight and obesity should be diagnosed using the body mass index BMI (your weight in kilos divided by your height in metres squared). Interpreting BMI in children is complicated because it changes naturally with age and differs between girls and boys.

BMI charts are available from:
* www.healthforallchildren.co.uk
* www.childgrowthfoundation.org

Facilitator Notes for Slide 7

Doctors use the body mass index (BMI) calculation to work out if a child is overweight. Although BMI has the potential to be distorting, it provides a convenient and accurate means of defining overweight and obesity in children. Although there is some concern that children might be misclassified or misdiagnosed when BMI is used, almost all children and young people with high BMI for age are excessively fat and many children not defined as overweight or obese using the BMI are excessively fat.

Activity Linked to Slide 7

Provide an opportunity for participants to share their experiences of BMI.

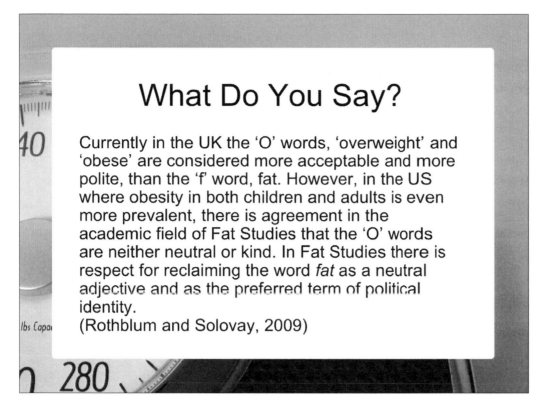

What Do You Say?

Currently in the UK the 'O' words, 'overweight' and 'obese' are considered more acceptable and more polite, than the 'f' word, fat. However, in the US where obesity in both children and adults is even more prevalent, there is agreement in the academic field of Fat Studies that the 'O' words are neither neutral or kind. In Fat Studies there is respect for reclaiming the word *fat* as a neutral adjective and as the preferred term of political identity.
(Rothblum and Solovay, 2009)

Facilitator Notes for Slide 8

In the US 'Fat Studies' is a radical, new field of academic studies that goes to the root of weight-related belief systems. Fat, in this context, is regarded simply as a descriptive term. Weight, like height, is a human characteristic that varies across any population like a bell curve. There have always been people of different heights and there will always be people of different weights. Fat Studies offer no opposition to what they regard as this straightforward fact of weight diversity.

Activity Linked to Slide 8

Ask participants to discuss with the person next to them, their reactions to the use of the terms overweight, obese and fat. Do they agree the term fat is less discriminating than obese or overweight?

Do participants agree that being fat is simply a fact of weight diversity?

Remind participants that the short-term consequences of childhood obesity are low self-image, low self-confidence and even depression and whether this is relevant to the discussion about the terms that are used.

Ask for feedback and discuss responses as a group.

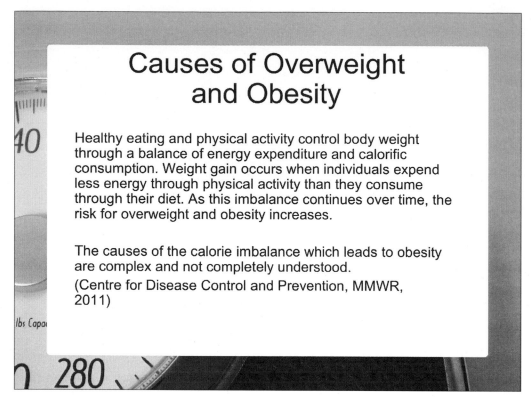

Causes of Overweight and Obesity

Healthy eating and physical activity control body weight through a balance of energy expenditure and calorific consumption. Weight gain occurs when individuals expend less energy through physical activity than they consume through their diet. As this imbalance continues over time, the risk for overweight and obesity increases.

The causes of the calorie imbalance which leads to obesity are complex and not completely understood.
(Centre for Disease Control and Prevention, MMWR, 2011)

Facilitator Notes for Slide 9

Weight gain is usually the result of a simple equation, more calories are being eaten than are burned off through exercise or other physical activity.

Studies have also established that sedentary behaviour in childhood and adolescence, particularly television viewing and other forms of screen time have contributed to the obesity epidemic. Sedentary behaviours are often linked to excess consumption of calories, exposure to food advertising and reduced feelings of satiety if eating while watching television.

Risk factors also include the consumption of sugar sweetened drinks.

An excess of high calorie food and a sedentary lifestyle pose a serious health risk. One common outcome is increased fatness. However, the identification of fatness as the problem, and resulting emphasis on weight loss and dieting is not the answer. It is important to shift the focus from fat and weight to choices leading to nutritional health and physical fitness, an approach that will enhance the overall wellbeing of the individual.

Activity Linked to Slide 9

Ask participants to discuss with the person next to them, their observations on the fact that an excess of high-calorie food and an increase in sedentary behaviour, especially 'screen time', has resulted in young people becoming obese and overweight.

Take feedback.

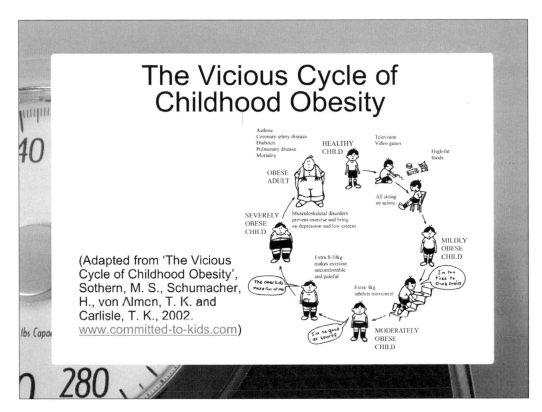

Facilitator Notes for Slide 10

The cycle of overeating, reduced physical activity and lower self-esteem will be to most practitioners, self explanatory and anybody working with overweight children could fill in the vicious cycle with more details of the ways a child is caught at each turn of the wheel. For example, teasing and bullying in the lunch hall leads to poor eating patterns and unhealthy food behaviours, hidden food, emotional eating and even binge eating.

In terms of physical activity, although many children get labelled as being 'lazy', it is their size that actually limits their active capabilities. Their extra weight results in reduced endurance and leg pain from stressed joints. Physical activity is demanding. Less ability to move, combined with reduced skills and confidence, results in continued weight gain as the cycle demonstrates.

Activity Linked to Slide 10

The cycle of overeating, reduced physical activity and lower self-esteem is self-explanatory. Ask participants for their observations on the cycle and take feedback.

Lead a discussion on how practitioners working with overweight children can help to break the cycle, for example, talking, engaging in artwork, writing a journal to enable children to deal with the pain that is inflicted upon them by teasing.

Ask participants to suggest some of the ways that overweight children feel encouraged, not embarrassed, during physical activity. Take feedback.

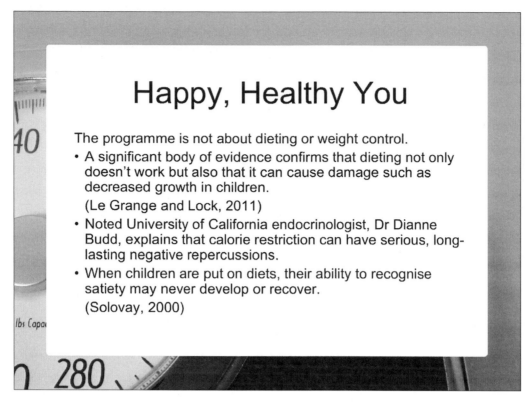

Happy, Healthy You

The programme is not about dieting or weight control.

- A significant body of evidence confirms that dieting not only doesn't work but also that it can cause damage such as decreased growth in children.
  (Le Grange and Lock, 2011)
- Noted University of California endocrinologist, Dr Dianne Budd, explains that calorie restriction can have serious, long-lasting negative repercussions.
- When children are put on diets, their ability to recognise satiety may never develop or recover.
  (Solovay, 2000)

Facilitator Notes for Slide 11

The programme is not about dieting or weight control. As a society, we have become so weight conscious that those who are treating obesity and eating disorders report seeing children as young as five years of age. Recent medical research, however, suggests that dieting is not an effective way to control weight and may actually have harmful effects. Low calorie diets are not generally recommended for children, as they can endanger normal growth and can result in children not being able to recognise feelings of satiety. A key message of the programme is that all individuals are lovable and capable just as they are, and that individuals come in small, medium and large sizes. Children's bodies will change as they grow.

Activity Linked to Slide 11

Children learn what is important to adults by listening to them and by watching them.

If children hear adults expressing dissatisfaction with their bodies, they may begin to believe that being an adult means being dissatisfied with their body. Similarly, when they hear adults being disparaging or critical about the bodies of others, they may mimic this behaviour by teasing other children about their bodies.

Think carefully about your own attitudes and feelings associated with your body and physical appearance before you run the programme in your class.

You may want to do the quiz which can be found at the end of Part One.

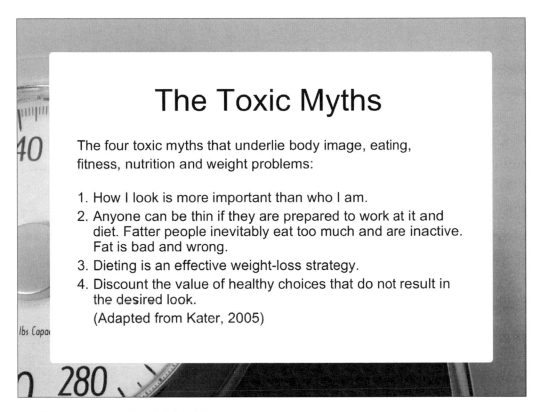

The Toxic Myths

The four toxic myths that underlie body image, eating, fitness, nutrition and weight problems:

1. How I look is more important than who I am.
2. Anyone can be thin if they are prepared to work at it and diet. Fatter people inevitably eat too much and are inactive. Fat is bad and wrong.
3. Dieting is an effective weight-loss strategy.
4. Discount the value of healthy choices that do not result in the desired look.

(Adapted from Kater, 2005)

Facilitator Notes for Slide 12

In producing a response to the current concerns about overweight and obesity it is important to recognise that the pervasive thin ideal, the diet mentality, poor nutrition and fitness habits and 'weightism' are all interrelated and part of the same problem. Solutions must therefore address all of these risk factors.

The Happy, Healthy You programme was designed as a response to the four risk factors that underlie body image, eating, fitness, nutrition and weight problems. Rather than teaching children what to avoid, the key messages of the programme emphasise what pupils can do to build positive living skills.

NB. The programme is not about dieting or weight control. Jenny O' Dea (2007) identifies that 'dietary restraint' during childhood and adolescence can have devastating effects on growth and development. It is therefore essential that facilitators refrain from talking to pupils about weight loss and dieting.

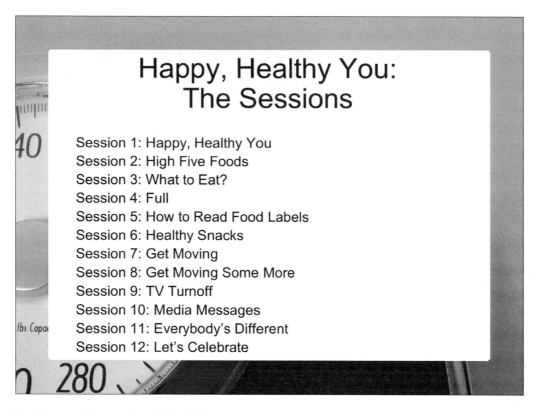

Facilitator Notes for Slide 13

This programme was written to provide teachers with an early intervention programme that can be used to explore with pupils what they can do to lead healthier lives. The programme consists of 12 sessions and focuses on key messages about healthy living that will not only help pupils to be healthier and happier right now, but will also provide the knowledge and skills they need for lifelong health.

Healthy living encompasses more than just eating a healthy and balanced diet. It also involves getting the exercise and rest our bodies need to stay healthy, as well as engaging in activities that we enjoy and that enhance our mental and social wellbeing.

Activity Linked to Slide 13

The programme emphasises a strengths approach to children building healthy living skills. The most fundamental way that we can do this is by demonstrating a healthy outlook on life ourselves, and committing ourselves to discovery of our own strengths and the strengths of others. Ask participants to discuss what a strengths approach and being a positive role model would mean for them in practice.

Take feedback.

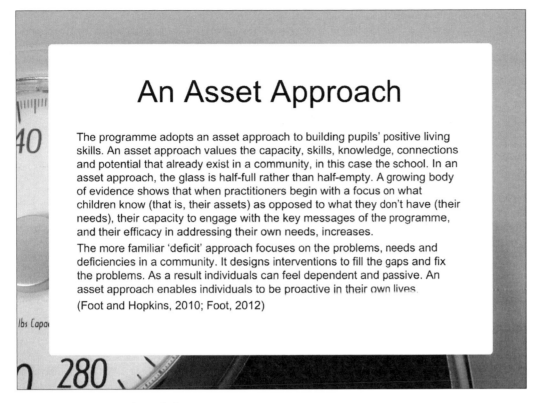

An Asset Approach

The programme adopts an asset approach to building pupils' positive living skills. An asset approach values the capacity, skills, knowledge, connections and potential that already exist in a community, in this case the school. In an asset approach, the glass is half-full rather than half-empty. A growing body of evidence shows that when practitioners begin with a focus on what children know (that is, their assets) as opposed to what they don't have (their needs), their capacity to engage with the key messages of the programme, and their efficacy in addressing their own needs, increases.

The more familiar 'deficit' approach focuses on the problems, needs and deficiencies in a community. It designs interventions to fill the gaps and fix the problems. As a result individuals can feel dependent and passive. An asset approach enables individuals to be proactive in their own lives.

(Foot and Hopkins, 2010; Foot, 2012)

Facilitator Notes for Slide 14

The shift from using a deficit approach to an asset based one requires a change in attitudes and values. Thus it is about celebrating pupils' existing practical skills and existing knowledge of positive living, their interests, networks and connections. The asset approach values the capacity, skills, knowledge, connections and potential in a community. It doesn't only see the problems that need fixing and the gaps that need filling. The more familiar 'deficit' approach focuses on the problems, needs and health damaging behaviours of individuals.

Activity Linked to Slide 14

Distribute the handout 'The Asset Approach' which is at the end of this section, and allow approximately ten minutes for participants to read it and discuss with the person next to them how they consider an asset approach would work in practice.

Take feedback.

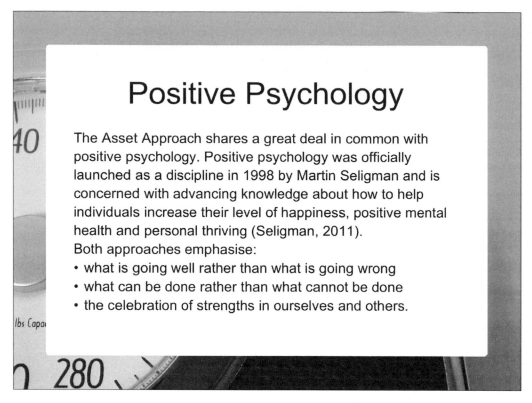

Positive Psychology

The Asset Approach shares a great deal in common with positive psychology. Positive psychology was officially launched as a discipline in 1998 by Martin Seligman and is concerned with advancing knowledge about how to help individuals increase their level of happiness, positive mental health and personal thriving (Seligman, 2011).
Both approaches emphasise:
• what is going well rather than what is going wrong
• what can be done rather than what cannot be done
• the celebration of strengths in ourselves and others.

Facilitator Notes for Slide 15

Before the introduction of positive psychology it was assumed that the absence of human adversities and troubles would result in human flourishing.

Thus if poor physical health caused unhappiness then good physical health would result in human flourishing. Positive psychologists have discovered that this is not the case, strengths have their own patterns, and health and flourishing is much more than the absence of misery.

Activity Linked to Slide 15

Provide an opportunity for participants to seek clarification on positive psychology.

Key Concepts from Positive Psychology

- Sonja Lyubomirsky (2007) discovered that each individual has a setpoint or characteristic level of happiness that is genetically determined and accounts for approximately 50% of each individual's happiness quota. According to this idea, we all inevitably return to our individual setpoint following disruptive events be they positive or negative.
- The happiness setpoint theory is similar to what experts have discovered about our weight. The weight setpoint theory suggests that we all have a healthy setpoint weight that is determined by our genes, metabolism and other factors, and is difficult to change. An individual may lose or gain weight but the body's natural tendency is to revert to its setpoint weight. With sustained healthy nutrition and levels of physical activity, it is possible to move one's weight setpoint down within certain parameters as with our setpoint of happiness it is possible to train ourselves to become happier. Seligman (2011) calls this 'learned optimism'.

Facilitator Notes for Slides 16 and 17

Unfortunately there is no laboratory test to determine an individual's setpoint, although scientists estimate that the average person has a setpoint range of about 10-20 pounds meaning that at any given time there is a 10-20 pound range at which your body will be comfortable and not resist attempts to change. It is possible to find your own setpoint by listening to your body and eating normally.

Distribute the handout 'Understanding Your Natural Weight Setpoint'.

Provide approximately ten minutes for participants to read the handout and then lead a discussion on the importance of encouraging children to eat naturally in response to signals of hunger, fullness and appetite.

Key Concepts from Positive Psychology (Cont)

Dr Linda Bacon (2008) founder of the 'Health at Every Size' movement suggests that it is helpful to think of our weight setpoint as the preferred temperature on a fat thermostat. The system then works hard to do anything it can to bring your body into alignment with that point. It acts like a biological force and the further you go from the centre, the stronger the pull is to get you back to the comfortable range. If an individual keeps 'jiggling' with the thermostat via diets, the mechanism breaks down. Your body then forces you to regain any weight you've lost. Rather than engaging in a battle with one's body it is important for everybody to achieve a healthy, natural weight.

Slide 17

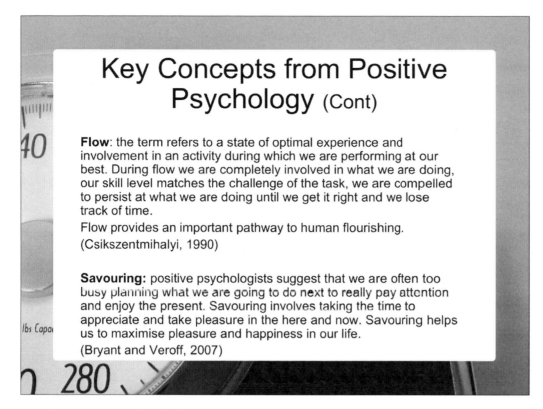

Key Concepts from Positive Psychology (Cont)

Flow: the term refers to a state of optimal experience and involvement in an activity during which we are performing at our best. During flow we are completely involved in what we are doing, our skill level matches the challenge of the task, we are compelled to persist at what we are doing until we get it right and we lose track of time.

Flow provides an important pathway to human flourishing.

(Csikszentmihalyi, 1990)

Savouring: positive psychologists suggest that we are often too busy planning what we are going to do next to really pay attention and enjoy the present. Savouring involves taking the time to appreciate and take pleasure in the here and now. Savouring helps us to maximise pleasure and happiness in our life.

(Bryant and Veroff, 2007)

Facilitator Notes for Slide 18

Throughout the programme, two key concepts from positive psychology are emphasised as being essential strategies for encouraging children to recognise that there is more to life than how they look. Encouraging children to explore a variety of activities which will bring them an experience of being in 'flow' and to take the time to savour the here and now, will enable children to feel good about themselves and appreciate their individual aptitudes and achievements. Learning to savour what we are eating is important. It is easy to see how not paying attention to food when we are eating may encourage us to eat more than we need. This is an important message with the current epidemic of obesity.

It is the inner feeling of worth that is generated by getting in touch with their strengths and abilities that will insulate children from anxiety about their looks and the need to conform to unrealistic ideals of physical attractiveness.

Activity Linked to Slide 18

Ask participants if they have ever caught themselves so immersed and absorbed in an activity that hours pass and they feel like they have been doing it only for moments.

Ask participants to share with the group the activities which enable them to achieve flow.

Ask for suggestions on how flow and savouring could both be encouraged in the classroom.

Take feedback.

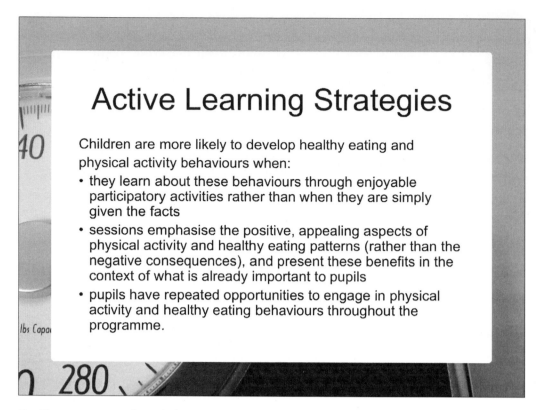

Active Learning Strategies

Children are more likely to develop healthy eating and physical activity behaviours when:

- they learn about these behaviours through enjoyable participatory activities rather than when they are simply given the facts
- sessions emphasise the positive, appealing aspects of physical activity and healthy eating patterns (rather than the negative consequences), and present these benefits in the context of what is already important to pupils
- pupils have repeated opportunities to engage in physical activity and healthy eating behaviours throughout the programme.

Facilitator Notes for Slide 19

When delivering the programme, it is important that teachers use strategies that are interactive and engage all pupils. This can be achieved by using demonstration, discussion and debate. Active participation in the programme will enable pupils to develop the concepts, attitudes and skills that they need to make healthy eating choices and be physically active.

Throughout the programme, pupils also learn how to make the connection between physical activity, healthy eating behaviours and their overall health. Developmentally appropriate strategies include, skill development, learning how to choose a healthy snack and self-monitoring (such as keeping a diary of physical activities and sedentary behaviours, tracking fruit and vegetable choices).

There is also an emphasis on self-assessment and setting personal goals.

Activity Linked to Slide 19

Provide participants with a sample session from the programme and allow up to ten minutes for each participant to read the session notes.

Give the participants an opportunity to ask questions and seek clarification on the content, structure and the practical aspects of delivering the programme.

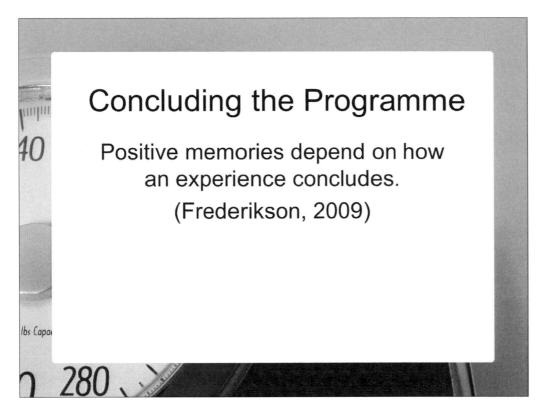

Concluding the Programme

Positive memories depend on how an experience concludes.

(Frederikson, 2009)

Facilitator Notes for Slide 20

Explain to participants that it is important to conclude the programme with a focus on 'what has gone well'. Positive endings, called 'peak end rule' by positive psychologists, create an overall positive memory of an experience, thus ensuring that the programme ends on a celebratory note and this will contribute to the overall effectiveness and success of the intervention.

Activity Linked to Slide 20

Provide a final opportunity for participants to seek clarification on any aspect of the programme.

Thank participants for their engagement and contributions to the presentation and wish them success in delivering the Happy, Healthy You programme.

The Asset Approach

The asset approach is a set of values and principles, and a way of thinking about the world. The approach:

- identifies and makes visible the health enhancing assets and behaviours in a community

- sees individuals, in this case pupils, as co-producers of health and wellbeing

- promotes relationships and friendships that can provide caring, mutual help and fun

- supports individuals health and wellbeing through self-esteem, coping strategies, resilience skills, relationships, friendships, knowledge and personal resources.

An asset approach starts by asking questions and reflecting on what 'assets' are already in place:

- What makes us strong?

- What makes us healthy?

- What helps us cope when things get difficult?

- What makes this a good place to be?

- What does the school do to improve our health?

In practice this means:

- finding out what is already working and generating more of it

- promoting more of what the programme is trying to achieve rather than focusing on what the problems are

- valuing the assets, as soon as individuals are talking to each other they are working on the solutions

- actively building confidence among pupils and staff

- involving all the class from the beginning, as those left out will be left behind

- ensuring the long-term sustainability of the project.

(Foot and Hopkins, 2010; Foot, 2012)

Understanding Your Natural Weight Setpoint

Are You Above Your Setpoint?

The following questions will enable you to consider if you are above your setpoint:

- Do you have difficulty recognising when you are hungry and when you've had enough?

- Do you routinely eat beyond a comfortable level of fullness and then feel lethargic, full and uncomfortable after meals?

- Do you go through times when your eating is out of control because you are intending to go on a diet?

- Do you skip meals in an effort to lose weight, then overeat because you are so hungry?

- Do you skip meals to 'save up' for a big feast?

- Do you often eat as a coping mechanism, for example, when you are tired, angry or nervous, or killing time when you're bored?

- Do you sometimes feel guilty about some of the foods or the amount of food you eat?

- Do you sometimes eat quickly without taking the time to focus on the food or savour and enjoy it?

- Do you fluctuate between periods of sensible, nutritious eating and then eat out of control?

If you answered yes to any of these questions you may be at risk of being above your natural weight setpoint. Don't feel bad. Most people aren't at their setpoint.

Health Warning

Many of these conditions may also be symptomatic of an eating disorder or other concerns. Be sure to discuss these symptoms with a trusted professional.

Understanding Your Natural Weight Setpoint (Cont)

Are You Below Your Setpoint?

Some individuals are below their setpoint. You'll know this if:

- you're often cold
- you feel like you're always thinking about food and often feel very hungry
- you wake up with an overwhelming urge to eat
- you have difficulty sleeping because of hunger
- you suffer from apathy, fatigue, irritability or depression.

If you are below your setpoint, learning how to respond to your body's signals will help you to normalise your eating habits and feel better. This may result in a healthy weight gain, but this is a good thing.

Health Warning

Many of these conditions may also be symptomatic of an eating disorder, a thyroid dysfunction or other concerns. It is important that you discuss these with a trusted health professional.
(Adapted from Bacon, 2008)

Research more about the weight setpoint theory at www.haesbook.com.

General Guidance on Delivering the Programme

This section provides practical guidance to practitioners on delivering the programme. It is written in two parts. The first part describes general information and the second part offers more detailed guidance on practical aspects of delivering the programme.

The programme that forms the backbone of this book has been designed as a structured, practical resource that aims to develop healthy living skills in primary aged pupils. Although the programme is a 'standalone' resource it is important that its approaches are incorporated into the daily life of the school. This is because the focus, healthy living skills, is directly about the pupils and being human, rather than being about more abstract ideas and facts. Teaching the programme is not like other academic disciplines because it relates directly to the experiences that pupils have in their daily lives and to just teach about these skills would be to miss the point. The programme focuses on healthy living skills and raising pupil's awareness of the influences that they are exposed to on a daily basis. The programme, therefore, must have experience as its main aim and pupil participation is a vital strategy for its success. The guiding principle for delivering the programme is that pupils should firstly experience the ideas and concepts for themselves, and secondly reflect and evaluate their relevance and usefulness to their own lives.

Teaching the programme involves a three stage process:

1.   Awareness and Noticing.

2.   Intervention and Action.

3.   Evaluation and Reflection.

Stage 1: Awareness and Noticing

This first stage of teaching takes place when the pupils are introduced to the concepts that form the programme. 'Noticing' is a primary skill because it is the alert system that tells us that things are going well or not going well, and the alert which lets us know that we need to make changes in our lives. It will be important to encourage pupils to be aware of their reactions to the material being presented in the sessions. Noticing and awareness arise from paying attention and these are skills that may have to be learned.

Stage 2: Intervention and Action

The programme is presented in 12 sessions. There is a developmental sequence to the sessions and it is most effective when they are delivered in the order in which they are presented in the programme. That said, in terms of the individual sessions, practitioners might decide not to complete every activity in each session. It is essential that the sessions are delivered flexibly, according to the needs of the pupils. Feedback from practitioners who have delivered the programme, suggests that pupils value the opportunity to explore ideas and engage in group or partner discussions, therefore, in terms of delivering the content of the sessions, less is more. It is more important for effective learning to take place rather than practitioners feeling under pressure to deliver all the activities suggested.

The facilitator should consider at the planning stage the needs of the pupils and the time available for the programme. It can be delivered to whole classes or to small groups. Signe Whitson (2012) suggests that young people do some of their best learning in small groups because they are more likely to feel supported by peers who are 'all in the same boat', and benefit from practising new skills with them. The bottom line is that flexibility is the rule as to how the programme should be delivered, and the needs of the pupils must be paramount if they are to benefit.

Timing of the Sessions

It is anticipated that each session will last for approximately forty five minutes and this should include plenty of time for group discussion and partner or individual work. The key criteria for effective delivery is that pupils feel that they relate to the content of the sessions and are able to complete the activities thoughtfully, based on their own experience, so they can:

- experience it
- put it into practice in their own lives
- reflect upon its usefulness in their lives.

Activity Pages

The activity pages which accompany each session are intended to be used as starting points for pupils' active involvement in the material being presented and to spark off responses based on their individual experiences. The importance of creating opportunities for the pupils to engage with the concepts that are presented in the sessions cannot be overstated. Unless children have time to consider how the concepts being taught can affect them as individuals, effective learning will not take place. Pupils may have an intellectual grasp of the programme's content, but the key messages of the programme will not, in Ian Morris's (2009) words, 'be embedded in the core of their being'.

The programme, therefore, allows for a flexible approach to delivery regarding time allocation. The bottom line is that practitioners should have the confidence and flexibility to deliver the programme in line with the needs of the pupils that they are working with. This may mean repeating a session or leaving out the activities to enable helpful and productive class discussion or partner work to continue. This flexible approach has important implications for the choice of the facilitator. The facilitator must be committed to delivering the programme and also:

- feel comfortable with the subject area
- be able to effectively engage with young people
- have a working knowledge of the concepts and strategies that form the programme
- feel comfortable facilitating discussions and provide a good model of listening to differing viewpoints without necessarily agreeing with them
- have a real commitment to developing healthy living skills.

Creating a Positive Group Environment

In order for the programme to be successful, it is essential that every pupil feels acknowledged, valued and able to contribute to classroom discussion. It will be important for the facilitator to model an open and honest communication style with the class and create an atmosphere where individuals are able to express their opinions, doubts and concerns without fear of being put down or that their contribution will be rejected.

Classroom management is more effective if classroom rules or guidelines are negotiated with the class at the outset. Making choices together, about how the class will be managed, is more likely to create compliance with the agreed standards. It may be helpful before commencing the programme, to spend some time working with the class on their classroom rights, rules and responsibilities.

Unicef UK has developed curriculum resources on rights and responsibilities for all phases of education: www.unicef.org.uk./education

Studies (Ryan and Deci, 2000; Thuen and Bru, 2009) suggest that pupils who perceive that they have a degree of autonomy in the classroom are usually committed and intrinsically motivated. They are more engaged in learning activities than pupils who perceive the classroom climate as being controlling.

Signe Whitson (2012) suggests that the facilitator can foster trust and create a positive learning environment by:

- role modelling positive and assertive behaviours in all interactions with class members
- demonstrating unconditional positive regard for each learner
- making learning pupil centred rather than teacher centred and giving pupils a say in setting their own learning targets
- conveying a belief in the abilities and skills of individual members and the class as a whole
- giving pupils structured opportunities to develop solutions to both individual and class issues
- differentiating and adapting the programme to the needs of the group
- actively encouraging participation by all class members
- providing individual feedback to pupils
- safeguarding pupils from put-downs and hurtful interactions
- asking group members for their opinions and feedback
- encouraging pupils to ask questions
- regularly celebrating group learning and successes.

Stage 3: Evaluation and Reflection

The third and final stage in the process is evaluation and reflection. This process should not be simply left to the end of the programme but should be an essential part of every session. Pupils should be encouraged to get into the habit of questioning the information that is presented to them and its usefulness. Pupils must be able to be open about aspects of the session that did not work for them, be encouraged to reflect on what could have been done differently and suggest constructive solutions. A key success criteria for the programme is that pupils feel able to reflect meaningfully on the effectiveness of the sessions as a whole for enabling them to develop healthy living skills.

Measuring Impact

As noted above, the aim of the programme is to introduce pupils to key healthy living messages and enable them to put these messages into practice in their own lives. This will involve:

- sharing the new learning with others
- actively using the new learning in their lives.

The impact of the programme can also be measured by whether the facilitator considers that, as a result of the sessions, pupils:

- notice things about themselves and the world around them and are aware of their internal alert system that lets them know when things are going well or not going well for them
- know the practical things and action that they need to take to keep themselves happy and healthy
- report increased satisfaction in their lives from using the positive living skills in their day-to-day lives.

As a result of the programme pupils should be able to have the following internal dialogue:

- I know when something helpful or unhelpful is happening in my life. I know this because...
- When... is happening in my life, I know that I have to...
- I know this is successful because...

(Adapted from Morris, 2009)

Involving Parents and Carers

When introducing the programme, it is important to inform parents and carers so that they understand its purpose. Staff should encourage parents and carers to talk to their children at home about the themes that are introduced during the programme. These discussions will support and reinforce the work that is being done in the classroom. Practical advice and guidance on how to include parents and carers is included in the concluding section of Part Two.

Guidance on Practical Aspects of Delivering the Programme

Scheduling the Programme

Whenever possible, it is important to schedule the session to take place at regular intervals. In my experience of delivering the programme in schools, weekly sessions are ideal, as this time frame encourages continuous learning and timely opportunities for re-inforcement. Pupils benefit from the predictability of knowing when the sessions will take place, and generally look forward to regular engagement in the programme. It is also important to avoid scheduling the programme for times when pupils will miss parts of the sessions. It can be exasperating for pupils to start addressing an issue but then not have the opportunity to finish it. It is also disruptive to the programme for the membership of the group to be inconsistent. When practitioners prioritise a regular time slot to deliver the programme, they signal to participants its importance.

It is also, as far as possible, important to select a single location for delivering the programme. The room should be large enough to:

- accommodate participants comfortably
- incorporate Circle Time activities
- allow pupils to move around the room during group and partner activities.

It is also helpful if the room is free from noisy distractions and that it provides privacy for participants to feel safe engaging in self-reflection and debate.

Delivering the Sessions

Length of Sessions

Each session in the programme can be delivered in about 45 minutes, although this time frame is offered only as a guideline and sessions may be extended (time permitting) or reduced, according to the size of the group. In our experience of delivering the programme, the larger the group, the longer the session is likely to take in order to ensure that it is interactive and that there are plenty of opportunities for discussion involving all pupils.

Structure of the Sessions

Each session, apart from the first and final session, follows a similar structure. However, it is important to emphasise that this is a suggested arrangement and the practitioners should feel free to adapt this structure according to the needs of their group.

Resources

The resources needed to deliver each session are listed at the beginning of the session notes. All activity pages can be printed from the CD-ROM.

Key Words

Key words are listed at the beginning of every session. These words are crucial to understanding the text and may have to be taught before the session so that the pupils' understanding of the concepts being taught is not compromised.

Aims

The aims of each session are listed in bullet points towards the beginning of the session notes.

Review of Previous Session and Take Away Activities

This component of each session is essential as the programme is developmental, each session building on the one before.

Introduction to the Session

The focus of the session is introduced to ensure clarity and to create a shared purpose for the session. They prepare pupils for learning using a framework or umbrella idea that provides scaffolding for the remainder of the session.

Right Now Activities

Pupils work on individual, partner or group tasks.

Review of Activities

Reviews take place through class discussion.

Take Away Activities

Follow up activities to extend pupils' understanding of concepts are distributed and explained.

Final Plenary

The aims of the session are reviewed and pupils evaluate the session using an appreciative enquiry approach of 'What Worked Well'.

Resources

In addition to the usual writing and drawing materials the resources listed below are required for delivering the programme. Specific resources are listed at the beginning of each set of session notes.

Programme Log

At the beginning of the programme each pupil should be provided with a Programme Log, an A4 ring file with dividers in which they can keep their work. A suggested format for the front sheet is included in Session 1. Pupils may wish to personalise this. A record form containing a list of the sessions can be found in Session 1. Pupils should be given a copy of the record at the beginning of the programme so that they have an overview of the sessions. Pupils can store this record sheet at the front of their Programme Log and update it after each session.

The purpose of the Programme Log is to enable pupils to build up their own folder of work associated with the programme. Pupils should use the Log to store their class work, 'Right Now ' activities and 'Take Away' activities from each session. It is very convenient for pupils to keep the resources from each session in one place as they are asked to refer back to earlier activities throughout the programme.

Pupils should be encouraged to take pride in their Logs and add to it their own personal thoughts and also cuttings from magazines and newspapers which are of interest to the pupil and relevant to the programme.

The Programme Log provides pupils with a vehicle in which they can ask the teacher questions about the sessions and to which the teacher can respond with comments, stickers and personal words of encouragement. Thus an important purpose of the Programme Log is to enable the teacher to have a more personal dialogue with each pupil about the programme.

Ideally pupils will spend a regular time each week on the activities that form the programme. In a classroom setting, a regular, scheduled time for pupils to work on the log can be very helpful.

Throughout the programme, literacy is emphasised as an active, dynamic and interactive social practice and therefore the use of drawings, cartoons, mind maps, partnership and group working is encouraged in order to explore concepts and complete tasks. Where children work in pairs or groups, each participant should be given a copy of the work produced.

It is important to ensure that pupils who experience difficulties with literacy and recording their thoughts and observations are not penalised in the process of developing their log. Thus, encouraging pupils to express themselves in a variety of ways is vital to the success and enjoyment of the programme. The availability of adult assistance to scribe pupils' views or help with spellings may be useful in some classrooms.

It is essential that the creativity and individuality of each Programme Log is celebrated.

Right Now Activity Pages

Each session has Right Now activity pages. These activities offer pupils opportunities to reinforce the skill or concept being taught. These activities usually require a small amount of writing or drawing and are completed individually, in pairs or in groups depending on the task. In most sessions it is suggested that the relevant activity page is enlarged to an A3 poster size and placed in a central position in the classroom so that it can be used as a focal point for the lesson.

Take Away Activities

Take Away activities are suggested towards the end of each session. These activities have been designed to promote a fuller understanding of the programme by building on and extending what has been learned in the session. Extension tasks are referred to as Take Away activities, in order to promote the basic message of the programme that the skills and concepts introduced should be practised in everyday situations. These activities have been designed to be engaging and relevant.

For pupils to be able to complete these activities they should not be distributed in the last few minutes of the session. Sufficient time must be allocated to ensure that pupils understand the tasks. Collaborative problem solving and enabling pupils to begin to think through the task in the session provides a graduated approach that can give pupils the confidence to believe that it is doable.

Devoting session time to explaining Take Away activities and collaborating on the first steps to completing them, explicitly communicates their significance, whereas rushing to assign tasks during the final moments of a session, creates time pressures that are likely to undermine pupils' confidence and understanding. Also, throwing in a task in the last few moments of the session gives the message that it is an 'add on' rather than central to the session.

Following up Take Away activities in the subsequent session is a must. Neglecting to follow up on tasks gives the message that they are not important, and by discussing and checking homework tasks, it is possible to celebrate learning, clarify misunderstandings and any other difficulties.

Partner Work

There are many ways in which pupils can be paired. However, whichever way the teacher chooses, it is important that pupils succeed easily in finding a partner. One of the most effective ways of pairing pupils is for each child to write their names on a piece of card or draw their own portrait and label it with their name before the first session. The teacher then distributes these name cards or portraits to each pupil randomly at each subsequent session or sets them out face downwards on a table for pupils to select, thus determining their choice of who will be their partner for the session. Pupils are able to select another card if they have previously worked with a child. Once pupils have 'found' their partner the expectation must be that they sit together and commence the activity in partnership. The need to be 'with' each other, rather than just sitting by each other, must be encouraged by emphasising positive body language and also effective listening and speaking skills.

Sometimes the teacher may decide to partner a particular pupil with a teaching assistant for an activity to enable the child to receive adult modelling of sharing and cooperative behaviour. In such circumstances it is important that the teacher removes that pupil's name or portrait from the class set, to avoid confusion when the pupils are selecting their partners.

Monitoring Partner and Group Work

It is essential that during the phase of the session when pupils are working independently or with a partner, the teacher provides vigilant monitoring. Visual and auditory scanning is key to effective classroom management. Firstly, the teacher can praise the pupils as they work in partnership with each other by identifying and highlighting good practice. Secondly, the teacher can catch problems early and assist pupils as necessary by encouraging reluctant partners, and being aware of partnerships that are likely to be volatile. This may prevent frustration on the part of some pupils and provide recognition and encouragement for their learning efforts.

It is useful if pupils conclude their time with each other in a friendly and positive manner. The overall success of the programme and its contribution to creating a positive climate within the classroom will depend upon the level of goodwill and cooperation that is shared by each member of the class.

Final Plenary

The final part of each session is the time when the teacher brings the whole class together to review the learning and also the cooperation that has taken place. Encouraging pupils to reflect upon their own learning can help them to identify steps of achievement as they occur. It is envisaged that pupils will increasingly value their achievements and enjoy a growing awareness of their learning throughout the sessions. By reflecting on their own work pupils can:

- enjoy a greater awareness of what they have learned
- understand the purpose of the sessions
- set themselves realistic goals
- enhance their self-esteem through pride in accomplishment.

The final part of each session is a time when the teacher can:

- provide an opportunity for pupils to share their work with the class
- lead a class discussion emphasising the main learning points which have emerged from the session
- review the lesson aims, allowing the class to consider whether they have been met.

It is important to finish each session on a positive note.

Confidentiality

As the programme is directly about the pupils, and being human, some of the sessions may raise sensitive issues. Pupils may feel vulnerable sharing aspects of their lives with others. It is, therefore, important that confidentiality is emphasised and established at the beginning of the programme and reinforced throughout the sessions. The general rule is that contributions made in the sessions should stay in the room. However, all those involved in the delivery of the programme must understand that if something is raised that indicates a pupil may be at risk, then the facilitator is obliged to report these concerns.

Child Protection

If the facilitator has any concerns regarding the safety of a young person, these concerns should be discussed with a senior member of staff and local safeguarding procedures adhered to.

Working with Parents

Parents often struggle with how best to address eating and weight related issues with their children. Many parents ask how they can help their children to have a healthy dietary intake, a healthy body weight and a positive self-image.

In working with parents a careful balance needs to be created between helping parents recognise the important role they play in shaping their children's eating behaviours, physical activity patterns and body image, and avoiding feelings of blame if problems do develop. It can be helpful to explore with parents the many layers of influence that impact on children's weight. Layers of influence include:

- children's individual characteristics (genetic dispositions)
- family influences, for example, weight related discussions at home and so on
- peer influences, for example, peer dieting
- school factors, for example, bullying policies
- community factors, for example, the presence of local fast food restaurants
- media messages.

Children's Individual Characteristics

Individual characteristics may include the following:

- Age. Children's sensitivity to being overweight tends to increase with age, with adolescents being most vulnerable.
- The child's sense of emotional wellbeing. According to research by Hill-Beuf (1990) the more vulnerable and insecure the child, the more likely it is that the child will be adversely affected by being overweight.
- Gender. Girls are likely to be more vulnerable than boys. However, this situation is gradually changing and Hutchinson and Calland (2011) suggest that there has been a significant increase recently in the number of boys who worry about how they look.
- Attitudes and behaviours to physical activity. Some children will naturally enjoy physical activity and have a positive attitude to regular engagement in sports activities. These children are more likely to respond positively to parental messages encouraging them to 'get moving'.
- Media use and messages. Frequent exposure to the media and especially to films, TV and videos featuring idealised images, is linked to lower self-esteem, stress, insecurity and negative moods.

Family Influences

Family influences may include the following:

- The pattern of family meals. A regular, daily family meal is generally recognised to be an important protective influence against a child becoming overweight.

- Parental engagement in physical activities. Parents provide important role models for their children. Parental enthusiasm for physical activity is catching. Parents who get moving are more likely to have children who get moving too.

- Weight talk at home. Parents who express concerns about their weight are likely to encourage their children to worry about their weight too.

- Family relationships and communication. Children who feel secure, loved and valued for their individual strengths are less likely to engage in emotional eating or eating for comfort.

- Eating out practices. The more a family eats at fast food restaurants the more likely it is that children will be overweight.

- Home food availability. In homes where there is sufficient supply of healthy food, children are less likely to resort to eating less nutritious food outside the home.

Peer Influences

Peer group influences are likely to include the following:

- Peer involvement in physical activity. Children who have a peer group who enjoy physical activity are more likely to engage in sports themselves.

- Positive peer group. A positive peer group that has a wide range of interests is more likely to influence the child to engage in a healthy range of activities.

- A peer group that is focused on body image and has a value system based on how people look, is likely to negatively influence the child to hold similar values.

- A peer group that is focused upon dieting will encourage the child to engage in unhealthy weight reducing practices.

School Influences

School influences are likely to include the following:

- A range of facilities to encourage children to engage in physical education and sports activities will have a positive effect on a child's willingness to get moving.

- The provision of nutritious school lunches and vending machines offering healthy snacks will support a child's ability to make healthy food choices.

- Weight-teasing policies. Schools that adopt a zero tolerance policy to teasing and bullying will support a child's growing confidence. On the other hand, widespread teasing and bullying will contribute to the likelihood that the child will resort to emotional eating to compensate for the pain of being emotionally hurt.

- Media literacy training. Schools that enable children to read media messages for what they are, reduce their susceptibility to commercial persuasion.

Community Factors

Community factors that can influence a child's wellbeing include the following:

- Access to parks, child-friendly recreational activities, walking and bike paths. The greater the access to these facilities the more likely it is for the child to engage in healthy leisure activities.

- Fast food restaurants. The more a child is surrounded by these outlets, the greater the likelihood that the child will eat unhealthily.

- Community. A cohesive community that offers opportunities for volunteer experiences and youth development programmes creates a sense of belonging and the child will be less likely to resort to unhealthy eating and sedentary behaviours.

Media Messages and Society Influences

In our society children and young people are under constant media pressure to look perfect and to judge their appearance against the images that they see in the media. When children feel that they are not matching up to this image they may judge themselves harshly and feel that they are failures or inadequate in some way. This can lead to unhealthy behaviours.

An analysis of these influences shows clearly, that although parents can play a very important role in influencing their children, there are many other influences that will also have an impact. This means that even if parents do everything 'right' children may still develop weight-related problems. It can be helpful to encourage parents to see their role as a 'filter' of the negative messages and a 'reinforcer' of the positive messages that may influence their child.

For example, parents can filter out negative media messages about the importance of a perfect body by limiting the use of magazines that contain these types of images. Parents can also avoid reinforcing harmful media messages by not talking about their own body dissatisfaction. Instead, parents can look for positive societal messages to reinforce, such as by pointing out successful family members and friends who have made important contributions in their careers.

Talk Less, Do More

Neumark-Sztainer (2005) developed four corner stones to help parents guide their children to develop healthy body weights and positive body images. An important aim of these cornerstones is to encourage parents to talk less about weight-related topics and do more to help their children feel better about themselves and engage in healthy eating and physical activity.

The Four Cornerstones

1. Model healthy behaviours for your children:
   - Avoid dieting, or at least unhealthy dieting behaviours.
   - Avoid making weight-related comments as much as possible.
   - Engage in physical activity that you enjoy.
   - Model healthy eating patterns and food choices.

2. Provide an environment that makes it easy for children to make healthy choices:
   - Make healthy food choices readily available.
   - Establish family meal routines that work for your family.
   - Make physical activity part of the normal family routine.
   - Limit screen time for watching TV and searching the Internet.
   - Support your child in getting involved in physical activity.

3. Focus on behaviours and overall health rather than on weight:

- Encourage healthy behaviours rather than focusing on weight loss.

- Encourage your child to develop a robust identity that goes beyond physical appearance.

- Establish a zero tolerance approach to weight and appearance teasing in the home.

4. Provide a supportive environment with lots of listening and talking:

- Be there to listen and provide support when your child discusses concerns about weight or appearance.

- When your child talks about appearance or being overweight make it a priority to find out what is really going on.

- Keep the lines of communication with your child open whatever happens.

- Provide unconditional love that is not related to how your child looks.

(Adapted from Neumark-Sztainer, 2005)

Strategies for Enabling Parents to Build their Children's Positive Living Skills

It is important for parents to accept what is not in their control:

1. Accept your own and your child's genetic predisposition. All bodies are programmed to be fatter, thinner or in between. Regardless of efforts to change it, over time all bodies will fight to maintain the shape they were born to be. Don't complain about your own appearance and don't share body concerns with your child. Don't make negative comments about your child's weight or appearance.

2. Understand that all bodies change developmentally in ways that are not in our control through healthy ways. You may be able to positively influence changes that occur at puberty, during pregnancy, the menopause or through ageing by making healthy life style choices, but these changes cannot be controlled. Focus your attention on what it is possible to achieve.

3. Listen to your child and help build your child's self-esteem. Teach by example and radiate a positive self-esteem and don't put yourself down. Teach your child to use positive self-statements. If you notice your child making a negative statement about themselves such as 'I can't do anything right' or 'I'm so bad at this' restate the comment in a more positive way. For example, 'You made a mistake this time but next time you will get it right'.

4. Eat well and satisfy your own and your family's hunger completely with wholesome, balanced, nutrient rich foods. Sit down together and enjoy regular family meals that include plenty of fresh, colourful fruits and vegetables.

5. Limit sedentary entertainment. Get moving and get your family moving with you. Emphasise fun and enjoyment. Everyone should develop a reasonable level of fitness and maintain it through life.

6. Understand that if you and your family eat well and sustain an active lifestyle, your optimum, natural weight will be maintained. Healthy, active bodies are diverse in shape from fat to thin and everything in between.

7. Have healthy, realistic role models who help you to feel good about yourself and encourage your child to choose healthy role models who are inspirational for what they have achieved and contributed to society, rather than for how they look.

8. Remember how you look is only one part of who you are. Talk positively about your child, recognising their skills and qualities, and offer reassurance about how they look. Encourage your child to develop a sense of identity that is based on strengths and talents and to express their opinions and celebrate their individuality.

9. Be media savvy and encourage your child to develop media literacy skills. Be aware of the hidden power of advertisements and educate your child about the strategies that advertisers use to make you feel that there is something wrong with you. Be alert to the information that your child is accessing through their computer and what they watch on TV.

10. Regularly tell your child that you love them and always will.

Example Letter to Parents

Dear

Happy, Healthy You

During the next term your child's class will be working on a programme called 'Happy, Healthy You'.

The aim of this 12 session programme is to build the children's self-esteem and confidence by developing their positive living skills. The programme will focus on encouraging children to make healthy eating choices and get moving. There will also be specific lessons on helping children to understand how the media, and particularly advertisements, can affect how they see themselves.

Throughout the programme your child will work on a variety of activities in the sessions and there are also activities that have been designed to be completed at home. Please read and let your child tell you about them.

A number of these activities involve gathering information from items such as food labels and advertisements. Please support your child in collecting this information.

Listening and encouraging your child to talk to you about the programme could be very helpful.

Your interest and involvement will ensure that the programme is successful.

If you would like further information, please contact me at the school. I would be happy to talk to you in more detail about this work.

Best wishes

Part Three: Happy, Healthy You Programme

Session 1: Happy, Healthy You

Session 2: High Five Foods

Session 3: What to Eat?

Session 4: Full

Session 5: How to Read Food Labels

Session 6: Healthy Snacks

Session 7: Get Moving

Session 8: Get Moving Some More

Session 9: TV Turnoff

Session 10: Media Messages

Session 11: Everybody's Different

Session 12: Let's Celebrate

Session 1: Happy, Healthy You

Resources

A4 ring folder with dividers for each pupil.

Flipchart/whiteboard.

Happy, Healthy You front cover, Programme Log and list of sessions.

A small piece of fruit or a raisin for each pupil.

Right Now Activity: Happy, Healthy Quiz.

Right Now Activity: Ten Key Messages.

Right Now Activity: Really Want to Do – Key Messages.

Take Away Activity: My SMART Goal.

Take Away Activity: Something New x 2.

Key Words

Physical, mental, social, nutritious, nutrients, accurately, acronym.

Aims

The session aims to:

- assess pupils' knowledge and behaviours related to the programme's key health messages
- introduce the importance of setting SMART Goals
- introduce the concept of savouring.

Introduction to the Session

This session aims to give pupils a concise overview of the programme and enable them to understand ' the big picture' of being healthy.

Whole-Class Introduction

This is the first session in a series of 12 in which we are going to learn about the different ways that we can help ourselves and others to become healthier and happier.

An important part of being healthy is being happy, enjoying ourselves, looking on the bright side and caring about our family and friends.

Class Discussion

Start the discussion by asking the class to suggest as many ideas as they can about what they think being healthy is and why it is important for us all.

The following questions should elicit a range of contributions based on personal experience:

- What is health? (Healthy body, healthy mind, belonging, having family and friends.)
- What are the things that make people healthy?
- Do you think that people can learn to be healthier?

Record pupils' ideas on a flipchart and display them in the classroom so that they can be referred to in future sessions.

In these sessions we are going to think about all of these aspects of healthy living. One of the important things that scientists have discovered is that our body and our mind work together. This means that if we look after our health, our body will work better and so will our brain.

If we work on our fitness level it will improve, we will become healthier and happier.

Right Now Activity

Happy, Healthy Quiz

This activity involves each pupil completing a quiz that assesses their knowledge of how to be healthy. Quizzes are an energising way to start a session as they are usually quick and fun to complete.

For younger children the quiz can be completed by the teacher reading the questions to the class and pupils responding by a show of hands. This information should be recorded, as it will provide evidence of the impact of the programme when similar questions are asked at the end.

NB. It will be important to emphasise that there are no right or wrong answers to the quiz. Everybody's ideas are important.

Allow approximately 15 minutes for the completion of this activity.

Ask pupils to share their responses to the quiz.

The purpose of this discussion is to:

- enable pupils to share their thoughts about health and thus expand their individual ideas about being healthy
- increase pupils' feelings of connection to each other.

It is helpful when a pupil volunteers a response to ask how many of the other pupils agree and had included the same or a similar point in their answer. Conclude the discussion by asking for any ideas that have not yet been mentioned.

Right Now Activity

Ten Key Messages

Distribute the handout, Ten Key Messages and explain that the ten key messages of the programme are that we should all:

1. eat balanced, healthy food

2. drink water every day

3. choose healthy snacks

4. get enough sleep

5. be active every day

6. work hard

7. have interests and hobbies that we enjoy

8. feel good about ourselves

9. understand that everybody is different

10. restrict television viewing and other screen time to less than two hours every day.

Right Now Activity

Really Want to Do – Key Messages

Display an A3 version of this activity page. Ask pupils to consider the key messages and think about the following:

- Are they doing some of these things already?

- What would they like to do more of in the future?

- Choose one goal that they really want to achieve now to make themselves healthier.

Suggest that pupils brainstorm suggestions for goals that they want to achieve.

Talk through with the class the different components of the diagram starting with the outside circle and working inwards. The final and innermost circle is the place where pupils should write down their key goal.

Ask pupils to complete individual copies of the Really Want to Do – Key Messages activity.

Review of Activity

Ask for feedback on the activity.

Explain that taking the time to write down your goals helps to make them happen.

Ask pupils to describe the healthy goal that they can introduce into their life before the next session.

Take feedback and scribe responses.

Take Away Activity

My SMART Goal

Encourage pupils to think through how they are going to set about building a new healthy habit into their lives.

Explain to pupils that when they are setting a healthy goal they should play it SMART.

Introduce the SMART acronym:

- **S is for specific:** make sure you know exactly what you want to do differently.

- **M is for measurable:** make sure you know when you have done what you have set out to do. Instead of 'I am going to walk more' write, 'I am going to walk to my friend's house every morning so that we can walk to school together on five days each week'.

- **Attainable:** Before you decide on a goal, think to yourself, 'Am I really going to be able to do this?' Think carefully, 'Is this a sensible goal for me to choose?'

- **Rewarding:** 'Is this something that I really want to do and will it make me feel happier and healthier?'

- **Time bound:** Be clear about when you are going to achieve this goal. Will it be in two weeks, in one month?

Emphasise that setting a SMART Goal is a way of achieving a personal goal.

Remind pupils that their SMART Goal action plans are intended to be working documents that can be revised or updated at any time. It is important to build in review dates so that you can see if goals are being achieved and when a new action plan is needed.

Take Away Activity

Something New x 2

Explain to the class that finding out about being healthier and happier is like a personal journey. On this journey they will each discover new things so it is important to take the time to appreciate these good things in our lives. Positive psychologists call this 'savouring'. Savouring means stopping for a moment and really enjoying what you are doing, using all of your senses.

Show pupils the Cadbury Creme Egg Advertisement. Go to www.youtube.com and put Cadbury Creme Eggs Ad (1985ad, 1992 Version) in the search bar.

Distribute small pieces of fruit to the class and ask them to savour each one and take their time to explore:

- how it feels
- what it looks like
- how it smells
- how it tastes.

Emphasise that taking the time to savour the things that we do increases our health and our happiness.

Ask pupils to take the time to really savour a new food and enjoy a new activity before the next session and to record this on the Something New x 2 record sheet.

Final Plenary

Reflect and Review

A Circle Time approach can be used to enable pupils to focus on the following:

- Ask pupils to take a few moments to think about what they learned in the session and then suggest a variety of endings for the following sentence, 'One of the things we talked about in the session was the importance of...'.

What Worked Well

- Ask pupils to share with the person next to them something about the session that they have enjoyed. Ask for volunteers to share their responses.

- On a scale of 1-5 (1 = not at all useful, 3 = quite useful, 5 = very useful) how useful do we feel this lesson has been? Ask pupils to do a high five if they thought the lesson was very useful. Ask the remaining pupils to think very carefully about the next question and invite their responses.

- What would we like to be different about this lesson if it was repeated for others in the future?

Happy, Healthy You

Name:

Class:

Happy, Healthy You Programme

Name:

Date completed:

Session 1: Happy, Healthy You

Session 2: High Five Foods

Session 3: What to Eat?

Session 4: Full

Session 5: How to Read Food Labels

Session 6: Healthy Snacks

Session 7: Get Moving

Session 8: Get Moving Some More

Session 9: TV Turnoff

Session 10: Media Messages

Session 11: Everybody's Different

Session 12: Let's Celebrate

Session 1

Right Now Activity: Happy, Healthy Quiz

Name: Date:

These questions are all about you. Everybody is different and so there are no right or wrong answers. Think carefully and answer the questions as accurately as you can.

Healthy Eating

Think about all the meals and snacks you ate yesterday from the time you got up until the time you went to bed.

Circle your responses.

1. Yesterday, how many times did you eat fruit?

    0   1   2   3   4   5   6 or more

2. Yesterday, how many times did you eat vegetables?

    0   1   2   3   4   5   6 or more

3. Yesterday, how many glasses of water did you drink?

    0   1   2   3   4   5   6   7   8 or more

4. Make a list of all the snacks you ate yesterday. Remember to include sweets, chocolate and fizzy drinks.

    •   •

    •   •

    •   •

Right Now Activity:
Happy, Healthy Quiz (Cont)

5. What time did you go to bed last night?

    What time did you get up this morning?

    How many hours sleep did you get last night?

                    6   7   8   9   10

6. Think about how active you are every day.

    I walk for .... minutes every day.

    I cycle for .... minutes every day.

    I climb .... stairs every day.

    I also: ....

         ....

         ....

Right Now Activity:
Happy, Healthy Quiz (Cont)

7. Think about the sports that you have played during the past week.

   Make a list of all the sports that you have done during the past week and think about whether they made you sweat and breathe hard.

Sport	This made me sweat.	This made me breathe hard.
....	Yes No	Yes No
....	Yes No	Yes No
....	Yes No	Yes No
....	Yes No	Yes No
....	Yes No	Yes No

8. Think about how much time you watch television after school each day (Monday to Friday).

   On most school days I watch television for:

   0-1 hour each day.   1-2 hours each day.   2-3 hours each day.

   3-4 hours each day.   4-5 hours each day.   5-6 or more hours each day.

Right Now Activity:
Happy, Healthy Quiz (Cont)

9. An important part of healthy living is building relationships with others. Complete the sentences about how you show you are friendly, caring, kind and so on:

- I show that I am friendly by...
- I show that I care about my family and friends by...
- I show that I am kind by...
- I include people who are not my best friends by...
- I have fun ideas such as...
- I forgive people when they upset me and get over it by...
- I have interests to share such as...
- I can laugh at myself and my mistakes when...
- I am a good listener because...
- I share when...

10. I care about how I look. Add some more examples showing how you care about how you look:

- I brush my hair.
- I keep my face and hands clean.
- I like to wear my favourite colours.
- I choose my clothes carefully.
-
-

The colour of my hair is:

The colour of my eyes is:

My hair is   Short   Medium   Length   Long   Curly   Straight

Overall, my size for my age is: Big   Average   Small

Another thing about how I look is:

Session 1

Right Now Activity: Ten Key Messages

Name: Date:

Eat balanced, healthy food.

Drink water every day.

Choose healthy snacks.

Get enough sleep.

Be active every day.

Work hard.

Have interests and hobbies that you enjoy.

Feel good about ourself.

Understand that everybody is different.

Restrict television viewing and other screen time to less than two hours every day.

Right Now Activity:
Really Want to Do – Key Messages

Name: Date:

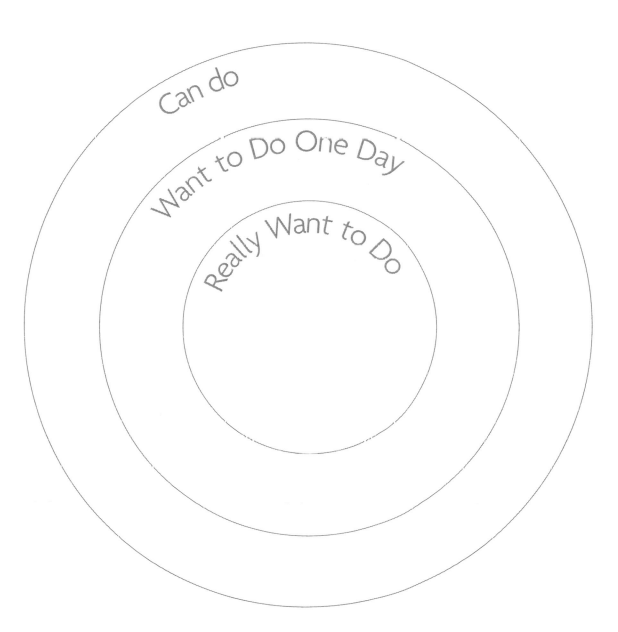

Can do

Want to Do One Day

Really Want to Do

Session 1

Take Away Activity: My SMART Goal

Name: Date:

Starting something new can be challenging and fun. Make a SMART Goal to help you achieve your dream.

My SMART Goal is to:

To make it happen think SMART.
All about my SMART Goal.

Specific. I know exactly what I want to achieve:

Measurable. I will know I have achieved my goal when:

Attainable. I can do it. I know my goal is possible:

Rewarding. What's in it for me? What will keep me working at this goal?

Time bound. Set a date. I will reach my goal on:

What help do I need to reach my goal?

How will I celebrate when I reach my goal?

Take Away Activity: Something New x 2

Name:

Week 1. Date:

Eat Something New	Do Something New
I tasted	This week I ....
....	....
for the first time.	for the first time.
I give it ..../10	I enjoyed it ..../10

Week 2. Date:

Eat Something New	Do Something New
I tasted	This week I ....
....	....
for the first time.	for the first time.
I give it ..../10	I enjoyed it ..../10

Week 3. Date:

Eat Something New	Do Something New
I tasted	This week I ....
....	....
for the first time.	for the first time.
I give it ..../10	I enjoyed it ..../10

Session 1

Take Away Activity: Something New x 2 (Cont)

Name:

Week 4. Date:

Eat Something New	Do Something New
I tasted .... for the first time. I give it ..../10	This week I .... for the first time. I enjoyed it ..../10

Week 5. Date:

Eat Something New	Do Something New
I tasted .... for the first time. I give it ..../10	This week I .... for the first time. I enjoyed it ..../10

Week 6. Date:

Eat Something New	Do Something New
I tasted .... for the first time. I give it ..../10	This week I .... for the first time. I enjoyed it ..../10

Take Away Activity: Something New x 2 (Cont)

Name:

Week 7. Date:

Eat Something New	Do Something New
I tasted .... for the first time. I give it ..../10	This week I .... for the first time. I enjoyed it ..../10

Week 8. Date:

Eat Something New	Do Something New
I tasted .... for the first time. I give it ..../10	This week I .... for the first time. I enjoyed it ..../10

Week 9. Date:

Eat Something New	Do Something New
I tasted .... for the first time. I give it ..../10	This week I .... for the first time. I enjoyed it ..../10

Session 1

Take Away Activity: Something New x 2 (Cont)

Name:

Week 10. Date:

Eat Something New	Do Something New
I tasted .... for the first time. I give it ..../10	This week I .... for the first time. I enjoyed it ..../10

Week 11. Date:

Eat Something New	Do Something New
I tasted .... for the first time. I give it ..../10	This week I .... for the first time. I enjoyed it ..../10

Session 2: High Five Foods

Resources

Flipchart paper and felt pens.

Right Now Activity: 5 a Day.

Right Now Activity: Foodoku.

Take Away Activity: NeverSeconds.

Take Away Activity: Something New x 2.

Key Words

Nutrients, infections, balanced, protein, treats.

Aims

This session aims to introduce:

- the concept of healthy eating
- the five main food groups
- everyday foods and sometimes foods.

Review of Previous Session and Take Away Activities

Remind pupils that in the previous session they were introduced to the key messages of being healthy and happy. Ask pupils to recall some of these messages.

Pupils were also introduced to the importance of writing down their goals and making them SMART. Ask for feedback and examples of goals that pupils have set for themselves.

Ask for feedback on the Something New x 2 activity:

- What new foods have the pupils savoured since the previous session?
- What new activities have the pupils enjoyed since the previous session?

Introduction to the Session

In this session we are going to be thinking about healthy eating. Healthy eating is just one aspect of healthy living but it is an important one because it:

- gives us the energy and nutrients our body needs to stay healthy and grow
- helps us to fight against infections
- helps prevent diseases
- helps our learning
- improves our mood
- is fun and enjoyable.

The foods we eat keep us healthy because they contain many kinds of nutrients. Nutrients are the chemical substances that our bodies use to build our tissues and organs and fuel our growth, learning and play.

The secret to healthy eating is choosing a mix of foods. This is because each group of foods gives us different nutrients. There are five main food groups to choose from:

1. Vegetables.
2. Fruit.
3. Bread and cereals.
4. Milk and dairy foods.
5. Meat, fish, eggs, nuts, seeds, tofu.

Ask pupils for examples of foods from each group.

Right Now Activity

High Five Food Groups

Divide the class into five groups, each group to represent one food group.

Give each group a large piece of flipchart paper and coloured pens on which they should write as many foods in their food group, that they can think of.

The group task is to think of more foods than the other groups and record them all on the flipchart paper.

After ten minutes each group should present their food poster to the class.

At the end of their presentation each group should ask for suggestions of any foods that they may not have included. A healthy diet will have different foods from each of the food groups.

Ask pupils to think about what they ate yesterday and whether they ate foods from each of the food groups.

Take feedback.

We should eat foods from the five groups every day and so we call them 'everyday foods'. The pupils can now complete the activity page, 5 a Day.

Right Now Activity

Foodoku

Distribute the activity page and allow approximately ten minutes for pupils to complete it.

Take feedback on this activity.

Right Now Activity

Sometimes Foods

There are also foods that we call 'sometimes' foods. All foods can have a place in a healthy and enjoyable diet but some foods are needed everyday and other foods should be eaten sometimes. Ask pupils to suggest what these foods may be.

Scribe their responses.

Explain that some people have an 'S Policy'. This means that they:

Treat Treats as Treats and have no Sometimes foods, no Seconds, no Sweets except on S days. That is, Saturdays and Sundays.

(Adapted from Pollan, 2010)

Ask pupils for their views on the S policy.

Take Away Activity

NeverSeconds

Review the NeverSeconds website. This blog is a daily story about one primary pupil's daily dose of school dinners. This site can be accessed at:
http://neverseconds.blogspot.co.uk

This site was created by nine year old Martha Payne. Martha calls herself Veg. Look at Martha's website and find out why. Martha blogs photographs of her school lunches every day. Her website has been visited by thousands of people.

Martha's blog shows that pupils can have a huge influence on their school lunches, so if you are not happy about your school lunch it's important to speak up.

What do you think about the website? Write a review.

Take Away Activity

Something New x 2

Remind pupils to eat something new and do something new before the next session.

Final Plenary

Reflect and Review

A Circle Time approach can be used to enable pupils to focus on the following:

- Ask pupils to take a few moments to think about what they learned in the session and then suggest a variety of endings for the following sentence, 'One of the things we talked about in the session was the importance of...'.

What Worked Well

- Ask pupils to share with the person next to them something about the session that they have enjoyed. Ask for volunteers to share their responses.

- On a scale of 1-5 (1 = not at all useful, 3 = quite useful, 5 = very useful) how useful do we feel this lesson has been? Ask pupils to do a high five if they thought the lesson was very useful. Ask the remaining pupils to think very carefully about the next question and invite their responses.

- What would we like to be different about this lesson if it was repeated for others in the future?

Right Now Activity: 5 a Day

Name: Date:

1. The most nutritious vegetables in no particular order are listed below.

Read the list carefully.

Put a tick next to the vegetables that you have eaten.

Put a circle around the ones that you enjoy eating.

Carrots	Avocados
Asparagus	Sweet potatoes
Broccoli	Peppers
Turnip	Spinach
Cauliflower	Peas
Brussels sprouts	Potatoes
Kale	Tomatoes

How many of these vegetables have you tasted?   ....

How many of these vegetables do you enjoy?   ....

2. The ten most popular vegetables are listed below.

Read the list carefully and number all these vegetables from one to ten.

Give your favourite vegetable ten and your least favourite vegetable one.

Tomatoes ....   Potatoes ....

Peppers ....   Green Beans ....

Cucumbers ....   Lettuce ....

Onions ....   Celery ....

Turnips ....   Radishes ....

Right Now Activity: 5 a Day (Cont)

3. Here is a list of the top 20 nutritious fruits.

Circle the fruits that you have tasted and give each of these fruits a mark out of ten for how much you enjoy eating it. If you enjoy eating the fruit very much give it a ten.

Papaya ....   Cantaloupe Melon ....

Strawberries ....   Orange ....

Tangerine ....   Kiwi ....

Mango ....   Apricots ....

Pink Grapefruit ....   Watermelon ....

Raspberries ....   Blackberries ....

Red Grapefruit ....   Peach ....

Pineapple ....   Lemon ....

Blueberries ....   Cherries ....

White Grapefruit ....   Banana ....

Keep a Look Out

If you do not recognise some of these fruits or vegetables, look out for them next time you go shopping.

- I found .... on ....
- I found .... on ....
- I found .... on ....
- I found .... on ....
- I found .... on ....

Session 2

Right Now Activity: Fooduku

Name: Date:

Fooduko is a puzzle using four food groups:

1. Milk and dairy
2. Fruit and vegetables
3. Grain products
4. Meat and alternatives

How to Play

In the grid make sure that each food group appears only once in the vertical and horizontal columns.

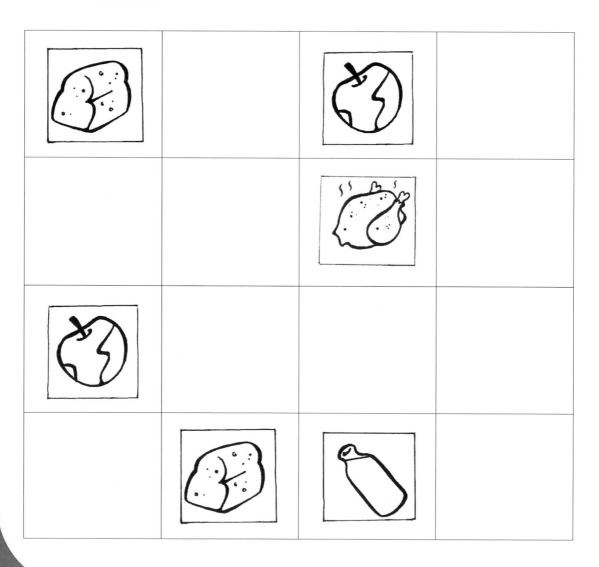

Right Now Activity: Fooduku (Cont)

	🍎	🍗	
			🥔
🍼			🍎

Take Away Activity: NeverSeconds

Name: Date:

Research the website http://neverseconds.blogspot.co.uk and write a paragraph about Martha and her school lunches.

Why is Martha called Veg?

What do you think about this website? Write a review.

Can you think of anything that would improve this website?

Session 3: What to Eat?

Resources

Copies of The Eatwell Plate. This is downloadable from: www.nhs.uk/livewell/goodfood/Documents/Eatwellplate.pdf.

Right Now Activity: My Balanced Eating Plan.

Take Away Activity: What to Eat?

Take Away Activity: Something New x 2.

Key Words

Balanced, nutrients, appetising.

Aims

The aims of the session are to introduce:

- the importance of eating a balanced diet
- The Eatwell Plate.

Review of Previous Session and Take Away Activities

In the previous session we learned about the five main food groups. It is important to eat food from each of the five groups every day because each one provides different nutrients. Choosing healthy foods gives us lots of energy and helps our bones and muscles to grow strong.

Ask pupils for the names of the five food groups and then for suggestions of foods from each of the groups.

We also learned that some foods are 'everyday' foods and other foods are 'sometimes' foods. Everyday foods usually have more nutrients, so it is important to eat them more often.

'Sometimes foods' have fewer nutrients so we should eat them now and again.

Remind pupils of the S policy.

Ask for feedback on the Take Away Activities from the previous session.

Ask for their thoughts on the NeverSeconds website.

Introduction to the Session

Ask pupils to think about the meaning of the word 'balance' and ask for suggestions that may include:

- being steady
- fair

- not falling over
- one side is the same as the other side, there is not a big side and a little side.

Ask for suggestions on how the idea of balance could relate to having a balanced diet.

The key point to emphasise to pupils is that having a 'balanced diet' means eating a variety of food from each of the five food groups every day. If you don't eat a 'balanced' diet and just eat one sort of food all the time, you won't get enough nutrients. Eating just a few types of food is not good for your health.

Introduce the Eatwell Plate

We can have a balanced diet by eating larger amounts of grains such as bread and cereals, fruit and vegetables and smaller amounts of meat, chicken, fish, eggs, and non-dairy sources of protein.

Right Now Activity

My Balanced Eating Plan

With a partner, work together and each plan a day's balanced meals and snacks.

Allow approximately ten minutes for this activity.

Ask pupils to review their partner's menu using the following scores:

- Foodometer rating, how appetising does the menu look? /10
- Estimate how many mouthfuls.
- Health rating, how balanced is the menu? /10

Ask for feedback on this activity.

Take Away Activity

What to Eat?

Ask pupils to keep a What to Eat? diary during the coming week.

Take Away Activity

Something New x 2

Ask pupils to savour a new food and have a go at a new activity before the next session.

Final Plenary

Reflect and Review

A Circle Time approach can be used to enable pupils to focus on the following:

- Ask pupils to take a few moments to think about what they learned in the session and then suggest a variety of endings for the following sentence, 'One of the things we talked about in the session was the importance of...'.

What Worked Well

- Ask pupils to share with the person next to them something about the session that they have enjoyed. Ask for volunteers to share their responses.

- On a scale of 1-5 (1 = not at all useful, 3 = quite useful, 5 = very useful) how useful do we feel this lesson has been? Ask pupils to do a high five if they thought the lesson was very useful. Ask the remaining pupils to think very carefully about the next question and invite their responses.

- What would we like to be different about this lesson if it was repeated for others in the future?

Right Now Activity: My Balanced Eating Plan

Name: Date:

Breakfast

- **Fruit** ....

- **Grain** ....

- **Dairy** ....

Morning Snack

- **Grain** ....

Lunch

- **Grain** ....

- **Grain** ....

- **Meat/Fish/Eggs** ....

- **Vegetable** ....

- **Fruit** ....

Right Now Activity:
My Balanced Eating Plan (Cont)

Afternoon Snack

- Grain ....

- Dairy ....

Evening Meal

- Meat/Fish/Eggs ....

- Grain ....

- Vegetable ....

- Vegetable ....

- Dairy ....

Take Away Activity: What to Eat?

Name: Date:

Keep a record of what you eat.	
Dinner	Other Meals, Snacks and Drinks
Sunday • •	
Monday • •	
Tuesday • •	
Wednesday • •	
Thursday • •	
Friday • •	
Saturday • •	

Session 4: Full

Resources

Right Now Activity: Full.

Take Away Activity: Finders Keepers.

Take Away Activity: Something New x 2.

Key Words

Influence, satiety.

Aim

The aim of this session is to:

- encourage pupils to explore some of the influences that affect their food choices.

Review of Previous Session and Take Away Activities

In the previous session we looked at The Eatwell Plate. This plate teaches us that we should eat different amounts from each of the five food groups every day.

Ask pupils for feedback on the Take Away Activities from the previous session.

Introduction to the Session

In this session pupils explore some of the influences that may affect their food choices. Ask pupils to look back through their What to Eat? diary and think about what influenced their choices of food.

The following questions may be useful to stimulate discussion:

- Do you think where you were or who you were with, influenced your choice of food and drink?
- Did how you were feeling influence how much you ate or drank?
- Do you eat more or do you eat less when you are feeling bored, tired, upset, lonely, angry, happy or stressed?

Ask pupils to brainstorm all the factors that may have influenced their food choices.

Four Key Influences

Introduce the following four key influences that affect how and what people eat.

Ask pupils to think about each of the categories:

1. **Who cooks and shops for you?** Who do you live with? What do other people like to eat and drink? Where do you meet your friends? What do other people want you to eat? Advertising? Holidays? Celebrations?

2. **How do we feel?** Hunger, thirst, taste, our likes and dislikes, our previous good and bad experiences of eating certain foods, our moods, boredom, eating or drinking when we are stressed, rewarding ourselves with food or drink, eating to please others.

3. **Price?** How much money do we have to spend on food?

4. **Religions.** Some religions require a vegetarian diet, some religions have strict food rules, some religions have special food on religious holidays.

Ask pupils to look at their What to Eat? diary from the previous week and think about whether their meals were influenced by any of these factors.

Take feedback.

Right Now Activity

Full

Explain that where we live can also influence how we eat:

- In Japan they have a saying 'hara-hachi bu' which means stop eating when you are 80% full.

- In India the Ayurvedic tradition suggests that you stop eating when you are 75% full.

- The Chinese suggest that you eat until you are 70% full.

- The prophet Mohammed said that a full belly is one that contains 1/3 liquid, 1/3 food and 1/3 air.

Ask pupils to choose one of these messages and create a poster to illustrate it.

Ask for feedback.

Create a display of the posters around the classroom.

Review of Activity

To say 'I'm hungry' in France you say 'J'ai faim', 'I have hunger' and when you are finished you do not say that you are full, but 'Je n'ai plus faim', 'I have no more hunger'. This is a different way of thinking about 'satiety' or being full up.

This week when you are enjoying your meals think about 'Is my hunger gone?'. This may happen before you feel full up.

Ask for feedback

Take Away Activity

Finders Keepers

Ask pupils to complete Finders Keepers where they have to find foods from different countries and identify foods with different characteristics.

Take Away Activity

Something New x 2

Remind pupils to savour a new food and have a go at a new activity before the next session.

Take Away Activity

Food Labels and Packaging

Ask pupils to collect labels and packaging from a variety of foods that come from different countries and bring them to the next session.

Final Plenary

Reflect and Review

A Circle Time approach can be used to enable pupils to focus on the following:

- Ask pupils to take a few moments to think about what they learned in the session and then suggest a variety of endings for the following sentence, 'One of the things we talked about in the session was the importance of…'.

What Worked Well

- Ask pupils to share with the person next to them something about the session that they have enjoyed. Ask for volunteers to share their responses.

- On a scale of 1-5 (1 = not at all useful, 3 = quite useful, 5 = very useful) how useful do we feel this lesson has been? Ask pupils to do a high five if they thought the lesson was very useful. Ask the remaining pupils to think very carefully about the next question and invite their responses.

- What would we like to be different about this lesson if it was repeated for others in the future?

Right Now Activity: Full

Name: Date:

Choose one of the sentences below and make a poster advertising its message.

- In Japan they have a saying 'hara-hachi bu' which means stop eating when you are 80% full.

- In India the Ayurvedic tradition suggests that you stop eating when you are 75% full.

- The Chinese suggest that you eat until you are 70% full.

- The prophet Mohammed said that a full belly is one that contains 1/3 liquid, 1/3 food and 1/3 air.

Take Away Activity: Finders Keepers

Name: Date:

One cheese from France is called:

One snack from India is called:

One rice dish from Spain is called:

One pasta fish from Italy is called:

Name foods from these countries and then find foods from some other countries:

Country	Food
Germany	
Japan	
China	

Which foods have these characteristics?

A vegetable that is purple:

A fruit as big as my head:

A cheese with a strong smell:

What is the most unusual food or meal that you have ever had?

Session 5: How to Read Food Labels

Resources

Right Now Activity: How to Read a Food Label.

Take Away Activity: More Food Labels.

Take Away Activity: Something New x 2.

Key Words

Ingredients, product.

Aim

The session aims to:

- understand how to read food labels.

Review of Previous Session and Take Away Activities

In the previous session we thought about some of the factors that influence what, when and how we eat. Sometimes we eat not because we are hungry, but because of how we feel, who we are with, where we live and how much money we have available to spend on food.

Ask for feedback on these influences.

We also thought about the ways different cultures think about hunger.

Ask pupils for feedback on the Take Away Activities from the previous session and discuss the packaging and labels that they have brought in.

Introduction to the Session

In this session we are going to try to understand more about the food we buy.

Distribute the packaging from a variety of foods so that the pupils can refer to them during the following discussion.

Explain that food labels can be confusing because there is sometimes a lot of complicated information on the label in very small print. Knowing the key things to look out for can help us to read the label and understand more about what is in our food.

Food Labels

Here is a list of the six main things that we need to know and can find out from reading a food label:

1. **Name.** Every food label names the food.

2. **Ingredients**. This is a list of what is in the food. All the ingredients are listed by weight so the first three ingredients are what the food is mostly made up of.

3. **Net weight**. This is the weight of the food without the packaging. Sometimes a lot of packaging can make the product look much larger than it really is so it is important to check the weight of the product rather than look at how big the item is.

4. **Nutrition panel**. This tells us how much energy in calories or kilojoules and how much protein, fat, carbohydrate, dietary fibre and sodium the food contains. Nutrients are usually shown per serving and per 100 grams. If, for example, a breakfast bar is listed as 35 grams of sugar per 100 grams, you know that it is 35 per cent sugar. You will also know this from the ingredient list.

   You can see how much fat is in the food by looking at the amount of fat per serving and the amount of fat per 100 grams. Anything below 3% is low fat, anything between 7-15% is medium fat and anything above 15% is high fat.

5. **Use by or best before**. This date tells us the time limit on the food. This is the date by which it is best to eat the food so that it does not go stale. It is illegal to sell food that has gone past its sell by date.

6. **Country of origin**. This is the country or countries where the food comes from and was made.

Right Now Activity

How to Read a Food Label

Ask pupils to work in pairs to complete this activity using one of the labels and the activity page.

Take feedback on this activity.

Take Away Activity

More Food Labels

Ask pupils to continue reading food labels at home and in the supermarkets during the coming week and to complete the activity page.

Take Away Activity

Something New x 2

Remind pupils to savour a new food and have a go at a new activity before the next session.

Final Plenary

Reflect and Review

A Circle Time approach can be used to enable pupils to focus on the following:

- Ask pupils to take a few moments to think about what they learned in the session and then suggest a variety of endings for the following sentence, 'One of the things we talked about in the session was the importance of…'.

What Worked Well

- Ask pupils to share with the person next to them something about the session that they have enjoyed. Ask for volunteers to share their responses.

- On a scale of 1-5 (1 = not at all useful, 3 = quite useful, 5 = very useful) how useful do we feel this lesson has been? Ask pupils to do a high five if they thought the lesson was very useful. Ask the remaining pupils to think very carefully about the next question and invite their responses.

- What would we like to be different about this lesson if it was repeated for others in the future?

Right Now Activity: How to Read a Food Label

Name: Date:

Draw a picture of the product in the large box and then read the food label and complete the other boxes.

| Product Name: | | Net Weight: |

| Main Ingredients:
1.

2.

3.

4. | | Nutrition:

Helpful information includes:

1.

2.

3.

4. |

| Use by or best before date: | Country of Origin: |

Your comments and observations about this packaging:

....

....

....

....

Take Away Activity: More Food Labels

Name: Date:

Choose three food products. Read the labels and identify:

Name of product and country of origin:
First three ingredients:
1.   2.   3.

Net weight:

Nutrition panel:

My observations:

Name of product and country of origin:
First three ingredients:
1.   2.   3.

Net weight:

Nutrition panel:

My observations:

Name of product and country of origin:
First three ingredients:
1.   2.   3.

Net weight:

Nutrition panel:

My observations:

Session 5

Session 6: Healthy Snacks

Resources

Right Now Activity: You Choose.

Take Away Activity: Traffic Light Snacks.

Take Away Activity: Something New x 2.

Key Words

Unsaturated, saturated.

Aims

The session will explain about the different fats that are in food including:

- unsaturated fats
- saturated fats.

Review of Previous Session and Take Away Activities

In the previous session we looked at food labels. These labels are important because they give us information about the food we eat. Food labels can help us to make healthy choices. Ask pupils for feedback on the food labels they have looked at since the previous session.

Introduction to the Session

In this session we are going to think about snacks. Our snacks are often 'eat in small amounts' foods. Snacks are important because they give us an energy boost and keep us going in between meals. It is recommended that children and young people eat three balanced meals every day and two snacks. This is because young people are still growing and during growth our bodies need energy and nutrients.

Ask pupils to make a list of their top ten favourite snacks or drinks.

Scribe their responses.

Suggestions are likely to include: fruit, sandwiches, ice cream, cake, biscuits, crisps, chocolate, chips, fizzy drinks, tortilla chips.

Ask pupils to suggest why some of these foods should only be eaten sometimes but not every day.

Suggestions could include that the food:

- may contain too much sugar that causes tooth decay
- may contain too much fat that is unhealthy for us
- can be filling and mean we do not want to eat at meal times

- can train our taste buds to only like very sweet or very salty food
- may contain a lot of calories that can make us fat
- are usually expensive
- may contain too much salt that is not good for us.

We can find out about what is in the food we are buying by reading the food labels.

Although most foods can fit into healthy eating, other foods especially those that are high in saturated fats, added sugar and salt should only be eaten sometimes.

Fat Facts

We all need a little bit of fat in our diet especially 'unsaturated' fats. Healthy fats help the body to absorb nutrients such as vitamins and minerals. We should not eat too much fat because our bodies find it hard to process and start to store it up.

Saturated fat is the unhealthy sort of fat. Saturated fat can build up in our bodies and lead to diseases. These are some of the foods to watch out for:

- processed meats like sausages and burgers
- butter and ghee
- cream and ice cream
- cheese
- pastry
- cakes and biscuits
- chocolate
- coconut oil and palm oil.

Unsaturated fat is a more healthy kind of fat and we need to make sure we have it in our diets. This is because it helps us to absorb vitamins and minerals. You can find unsaturated fat in:

- avocados
- nuts and seeds
- sunflower oil
- olive oil
- vegetable oil
- spreads made from vegetable oils.

Sugar

There are lots of different words for sugar. Here are some of them:

- glucose
- sucrose
- fructose
- maltose
- corn syrup.

Remind pupils that we can find out about what is in snacks we buy by reading the food label. Ask pupils to suggest what information they should look out for?

Right Now Activity

You Choose

The children have to complete an activity where they have to identify the most healthy food choice and do a word search to find the different types of sugar.

Review of Activity

Take feedback.

Take Away Activity

Traffic Light Snacks

The activity requires the children to keep a record of the type of snacks they eat in the course of the week.

Take Away Activity

Something New x 2

Encourage the children to keep trying new foods and activities. It might be a good time to revisit the meaning of 'savour'.

Final Plenary

Reflect and Review

A Circle Time approach can be used to enable pupils to focus on the following:

- Ask pupils to take a few moments to think about what they learned in the session and then suggest a variety of endings for the following sentence, 'One of the things we talked about in the session was the importance of...'.

What Worked Well

- Ask pupils to share with the person next to them something about the session that they have enjoyed. Ask for volunteers to share their responses.

- On a scale of 1-5 (1 = not at all useful, 3 = quite useful, 5 = very useful) how useful do we feel this lesson has been? Ask pupils to do a high five if they thought the lesson was very useful. Ask the remaining pupils to think very carefully about the next question and invite their responses.

- What would we like to be different about this lesson if it was repeated for others in the future?

Right Now Activity: You Choose

Name: Date:

1. Choose the healthier snack choice in each of the boxes below:

Ice cream	Fresh apples slices	Crisps
Low-fat frozen yoghurt	Apple pie	Pretzels

Chocolate milkshake.	Oven baked chips	Sausages
Low fat chocolate milk	French fries	Skinless chicken

Hamburger	Cottage cheese	Nuts
Grilled fish finger	Cream cheese	Hot dog

2. Sugar Search
There are a lot of different names for sugar: glucose, sucrose, fructose, maltose and corn syrup. Find them in the word search below.

A	P	M	N	Z	W	Y	Q	M	L	H	J	Y
Z	O	N	P	Q	V	N	E	A	I	E	B	C
Z	W	Y	I	N	K	F	L	L	F	T	H	P
C	D	E	F	Z	Y	R	K	T	I	U	R	E
Z	A	T	P	M	G	U	Q	O	P	R	S	T
H	O	L	G	L	U	C	O	S	E	Y	D	M
F	Z	W	C	B	M	T	O	E	O	F	R	G
X	N	F	T	E	I	O	M	B	C	G	H	L
W	Z	C	O	R	N	S	Y	R	U	P	H	L
S	U	C	R	O	S	E	B	C	P	U	F	G

Take Away Activity: Traffic Light Snacks

Name: Date:

Here is a list of the top five Green Light Snacks, Amber Light Snacks and Red Light Snacks.

Green Light Snacks are low in fat and sugar, have lots of nutrients and can be eaten every day.

1. Fresh sliced vegetables with low fat dip.

2. 100% fruit juice ice lollies.

3. Non-fat plain yogurt with a teaspoon of jam or fresh fruit.

4. Whole grain bread, toast or rolls spread thinly with peanut butter or jam.

5. Baked potato with low fat cheese.

Amber Light Snacks have a smaller amount of fat and sugar and can be eaten two or three times every week.

1. Oatmeal biscuits, fig bars.

2. Non-fat frozen yogurt.

3. Potato salad, pasta salad, bean salad, coleslaw.

4. Nuts.

5. Granola bars.

Red Light Snacks have a lot of fat and sugar, eat once a week or less.

1. Cake, doughnuts, biscuits, cupcakes.

2. Crisps, cheese puffs, tortilla chips.

3. French fries, onion rings.

4. Ice cream, ice cream bars.

5. Chocolate, sweets.

Session 6

Take Away Activity:
Traffic Light Snacks (Cont)

Keep a record of the snacks you eat over the next week.
Colour each square red, amber or green depending on what sort of snack you have eaten.

Monday				
Tuesday				
Wednesday				
Thursday				
Friday				
Saturday				
Sunday				

This week I have eaten:

.... Green Light Snacks.

.... Amber Light Snacks.

.... Red Light Snacks.

Read about '2 Snacks Max' at the www.eatwell.gov.uk.

Session 7: Get Moving

Resources

Right Now Activity: Run Puppy, Run.

Take Away Activity: My Activity Diary.

Take Away Activity: Something New x 2.

Key Words

Sedentary, sluggish, kennel.

Aim

The aim of this session is to:

- teach pupils the importance of physical activity for healthy living.

Review of Previous Session and Take Away Activities

In the previous session we looked at different sorts of snacks. Growing children need to eat snacks and it is important to think about the sort of snacks that we are eating. Ask pupils for examples of green, amber and red traffic light snacks.

Reading food labels can help us to find out what is in the snacks that we choose.

Every one of the five food groups can provide healthy snacks.

Introduction to the Session

Healthy, happy living involves not only eating well and having a varied and balanced diet, it is also about how we spend our time. A balanced lifestyle means enjoying doing a variety of activities. Ask pupils to brainstorm what some of these activities may be.

Possible suggestions could include:

- spending time with friends
- talking with family members
- listening to music
- dancing
- jogging
- running
- playing sports.

Scribe pupils' responses as one of the aims of the discussion is to encourage all pupils to recognise that there are a variety of new and different activities to enjoy.

Right Now Activity

Favourite Activities

This activity should take approximately five minutes.

Ask pupils to work with a partner and spend two minutes each, talking about their favourite activity. Each pupil should select a different activity.

Take feedback and ask pupils how they felt when they were talking about their favourite activity.

As the aim of this excercise is to capture pupils' enthusiasm and enjoyment, it will be important to scribe the positive words and phrases that pupils use during this partner work.

Discussion

Explain that some time ago people had to do a great deal of hard physical work every day. They had to work hard to keep their houses clean, to get around and to gather their food and water. They did not have to think about making time for exercise. Their lives were already full of exercise just to get through the day.

Today, we have a lot of machines to help us to do housework and we have transport to help us to get around. This means that we can go through our lives without doing the physical activity that our bodies need to keep them strong, fit and healthy. We also have new ways to spend our time that involve us sitting down. People spend more time sitting down or being sedentary than ever before. Too much sitting down can make us sluggish. It is also harder to use the energy in the food we eat if we are not active.

Ask pupils for their comments.

Too much sitting down and being sedentary is not good for us. Muscles that are not well used, such as our heart, lungs, legs and arms become weak. When this happens, our heart has to work much harder to circulate the blood that keeps our body working properly. This means that we are more at risk of developing diseases.

We know we are exercising the muscles of our heart and lungs when we move our arms and legs until we are breathing hard and our heart is pumping faster than normal.

Right Now Activity

Physical Exercise

Ask pupils to stand by their desks or alternatively, if possible, do this activity in the playground. Ask pupils to run or hop while moving their arms up and down rhythmically above their heads until they begin to feel that they are breathing hard and that their hearts are pumping.

NB. For some pupils this will happen very quickly and for others it may take a few minutes. The more physically fit one is, the longer this takes in most cases. The purpose of this activity is for pupils to consciously experience the point at which their heart and lungs begin to work harder.

Ask pupils to imagine that they have been given a playful, young puppy. The puppy has been kept in a nice kennel and been given healthy food since it was born, but the puppy is not used to getting any exercise. The puppy has never gone for walks or runs and has had to stay in the kennel inside the owner's house every day. The puppy has grown very weak and does not know how to run and jump about.

Now that you are the new owner what will you do to make sure that the puppy knows how to run and jump so that he will grow healthy and strong? How do you think the dog will feel? How will the dog behave?

Right Now Activity

Run, Puppy, Run

Create a storyboard of drawings and sentences to tell the story of how you taught your puppy to run.

Review of Activity

Emphasise to pupils that being physically active every day makes us healthier, stronger and happier. It can also help to make our intelligence grow.

Take Away Activity

My Activity Diary

Ask pupils to keep an activity diary for the next week that includes naming the activity and the amount of time spent doing it. Have a discussion about what 'active' means.

Take Away Activity

Something New x 2

Encourage the children to keep trying new foods and activities.

Final Plenary

Reflect and Review

A Circle Time approach can be used to enable pupils to focus on the following:

- Ask pupils to take a few moments to think about what they learned in the session and then suggest a variety of endings for the following sentence, 'One of the things we talked about in the session was the importance of...'.

What Worked Well

- Ask pupils to share with the person next to them something about the session that they have enjoyed. Ask for volunteers to share their responses.

- On a scale of 1-5 (1 = not at all useful, 3 = quite useful, 5 = very useful) how useful do we feel this lesson has been? Ask pupils to do a high five if they thought the lesson was very useful. Ask the remaining pupils to think very carefully about the next question and invite their responses.

- What would we like to be different about this lesson if it was repeated for others in the future?

Right Now Activity: Run, Puppy, Run

Name: Date:

In the boxes below, write and draw your story of how you encouraged your puppy to run. Give your puppy a name and remember that in the beginning the puppy had been kept in nice kennel and given healthy food to eat but was not used to getting any exercise.

The puppy is called:

1.	2.
3.	4.
5.	6.

141

Take Away Activity: My Activity Diary

Name: Date:

In the boxes, write what the activity was and approximately how long you spent doing it. At the end of the day, write in the total activity time.

	Activity 1	Activity 2	Activity 3	Activity 4	Activity 5	Total Time
Monday	Time:	Time:	Time:	Time:	Time:	
Tuesday	Time:	Time:	Time:	Time:	Time:	
Wednesday	Time:	Time:	Time:	Time:	Time:	
Thursday	Time:	Time:	Time:	Time:	Time:	
Friday	Time:	Time:	Time:	Time:	Time:	
Saturday	Time:	Time:	Time:	Time:	Time:	
Sunday	Time:	Time:	Time:	Time:	Time:	

Session 8: Get Moving Some More

Resources

Right Now Activity: My Free Time.

Take Away Activity: Get Moving.

Take Away Activity: Something New x 2.

Key Words

Pyramid, category.

Aims

The aims of the session are to:

- introduce the categories of movement
- reinforce the importance of being physically active everyday.

Review of Previous Session and Take Away Activities

The previous session introduced pupils to the importance of being physically active for our health, wellbeing and happiness.

Ask pupils for feedback on the Activity Diaries that they have kept since the previous session.

Check on Something New x 2 and take feedback on things that the pupils have been savouring and new activities they have been doing.

Introduction to the Session

Explain the five categories of movement:

1. **Passive sitting (sedentary)**. Awake but sitting still.
2. **Active sitting**. Sitting with the upper body busy.
3. **Everyday movement**. Everyday movement on your feet.
4. Vigorous movement. On the go at a faster pace.
5. **Aerobic movement**. Working large muscles so the heart is beating quickly for more than 15 minutes.

Organise pupils to work in five groups. Give each group a category of movement and ask them to brainstorm some examples of the movements that fit into that category. Allow approximately ten minutes for this activity.

Ask each of the five groups for feedback.

Discussion

Ask pupils to think about their Activity Diaries for the previous week and answer the following questions:

- Did you get plenty of everyday movement each day?
- Did you get vigorous movement everyday?
- What do you think about the amount of time that you spent sitting during your days?
- Do you think that you're getting enough physical activity?

Ask pupils how they can fit more activity into their lives.

Emphasise the importance of thinking about their daily free time choices, before school and after school and use these as times to get moving. This may mean actively looking for opportunities to move, walking instead of getting a lift, climbing stairs instead of using the escalator or lift, walking to see a friend rather than sending a text.

Encourage pupils to set realistic goals for what they can do to get moving every day.

Explain that pupils also need to plan their time so that they can include activities and sports that involve more vigorous and energetic movement.

Emphasise the importance of choosing sports and activities that they enjoy and will look forward to being involved in.

Right Now Activity

My Free Time

This excercise involves pupils completing the activity page with examples of the different categories of movement that they engage in (adapted from Kater 2005).

Take feedback ensuring that pupils understand the five categories of movement.

Take Away Activity

Get Moving

Ask pupils to keep an Activity Diary over the coming week that records how much time they spend involved in the five categories of movement.

Take Away Activity

Something New x 2

Remind the children to keep savouring new foods and enjoying new activities.

Final Plenary

Reflect and Review

A Circle Time approach can be used to enable pupils to focus on the following:

- Ask pupils to take a few moments to think about what they learned in the session and then suggest a variety of endings for the following sentence, 'One of the things we talked about in the session was the importance of…'.

What Worked Well

- Ask pupils to share with the person next to them something about the session that they have enjoyed. Ask for volunteers to share their responses.

- On a scale of 1-5 (1 = not at all useful, 3 = quite useful, 5 = very useful) how useful do we feel this lesson has been? Ask pupils to do a high five if they thought the lesson was very useful. Ask the remaining pupils to think very carefully about the next question and invite their responses.

- What would we like to be different about this lesson if it was repeated for others in the future?

Right Now Activity: My Free Time

Name: Date:

Fill in the boxes to show what you do in the five categories of movement:

---

1. Passive Sitting

-
-
-
-

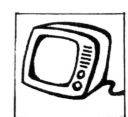

For example, TV, reading.

---

2. Active Sitting

-
-
-
-

For example, drawing a picture, writing.

---

3. Everyday Movement

-
-
-
-

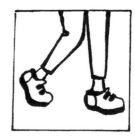

For example, walking, making your bed.

Right Now Activity: My Free Time (Cont)

Name: Date:

Fill in the boxes to show what you do in the five categories of movement:

---

4. Vigorous Movement

-

-

-

-

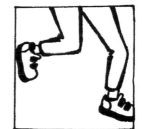

For example, on the go, jogging.

---

5. Aerobic Movement

-

-

-

-

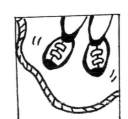

For example, the heart beats quickly, running, swimming.

Take Away Activity: Get Moving

Name: Date:

Complete the chart for each day showing the five categories of movement. Write down what activity you did.

	Passive Sitting	Active Sitting	Everyday Movement	Vigorous Movement	Aerobic Movement
Monday					
Tuesday					
Wednesday					
Thursday					
Friday					
Saturday					
Sunday					

Session 9: TV Turnoff

Resources

Right Now Activity: Screen Time.

Right Now Activity: Instead of Watching Television I Could...

Take Away Activity: My Fit Prime Time.

Take Away Activity: Something New x 2.

Key Words

Prime time, sedentary.

Aims:

This session aims to:

- enable pupils to be aware of the amount of time they spend watching television
- encourage pupils to consider healthy alternatives to watching television, particularly choices that involve more physical activity.

Review of Previous Session and Take Away Activities

The previous session introduced the five categories of movement. Ask pupils to feed back on the extent to which they have engaged in each of the five categories since the previous session.

Introduction to the Session

Explain to pupils that studies suggest that young people on average watch four hours of television each day. Most of this television is watched during 'prime time'. Ask children what they think is 'prime time' for watching television?

Clarify that prime time television is between 4pm and 9pm each day. This is the time when many people, especially children, are watching television.

Ask pupils to identify the favourite shows that they watch between 4pm and 9pm each day. Scribe pupils' responses and list the programmes in order starting with the most favourite programme, the second favourite programme and so on.

Watching less TV is better. Doctors recommend that children watch no more than two hours of television or video each day.

Explain to pupils that the more television that they watch, the less time they have to get moving and the less time they have to socialise with family and friends. The same goes for all screen time, such as surfing the web, text messaging and playing video games.

Right Now Activity

Screen Time

Ask pupils to complete the graph to represent their TV viewing hours and also the time that they spend surfing the web, text messaging and playing PC and video games in a named day.

Discussion

Emphasise to pupils that watching less than two hours screen time every day can help them to get fit.

Being inactive every day for more than two hours can make you lose flexibility, muscle strength and mean that your heart and lungs don't work so efficiently.

When you sit still, you burn fewer calories than when you get moving.

Also, watching television may mean that you eat more snacks and watch lots of advertisements.

Ask pupils for suggestions as to how they could cut down on TV and screen time.

Suggestions may include:

- watch only the shows and films that you really enjoy
- if you find yourself just sitting watching television and not really enjoying it, get moving and do something that is more fun
- spend time with a friend
- help your family instead.

Ask pupils to suggest what programmes they would choose to stop watching so that they could do other things and join in more activities. Ensure that this suggestion also includes pupils who do not watch prime time television but could engage in more physical activity.

Right Now Activity

Instead of Watching TV I Could...

Ask pupils to record on the activity page what activities they could participate in when not watching television (both physical activities and mental activities).

Review of Activity

Take feedback and encourage the pupils to make some of these suggestions happen.

Take Away Activity

My Fit Prime Time

Ask pupils to keep a record over the coming week of the times that they chose not to watch prime time television and engage in a different activity instead.

Take Away Activity

Newspapers and Magazines

Ask pupils to collect a variety of advertisements from magazines or newspapers and bring them to the next session.

Take Away Activity

Something New x 2

Pupils should try some new food and enjoy a new activity.

Final Plenary

Reflect and Review

A Circle Time approach can be used to enable pupils to focus on the following:

- Ask pupils to take a few moments to think about what they learned in the session and then suggest a variety of endings for the following sentence, 'One of the things we talked about in the session was the importance of...'.

What Worked Well

- Ask pupils to share with the person next to them something about the session that they have enjoyed. Ask for volunteers to share their responses.

- On a scale of 1-5 (1 = not at all useful, 3 = quite useful, 5 = very useful) how useful do we feel this lesson has been? Ask pupils to do a high five if they thought the lesson was very useful. Ask the remaining pupils to think very carefully about the next question and invite their responses.

- What would we like to be different about this lesson if it was repeated for others in the future?

Right Now Activity: Screen Time

Name: Date:

Draw a graph to indicate how much time you spent looking at a screen.

Day:

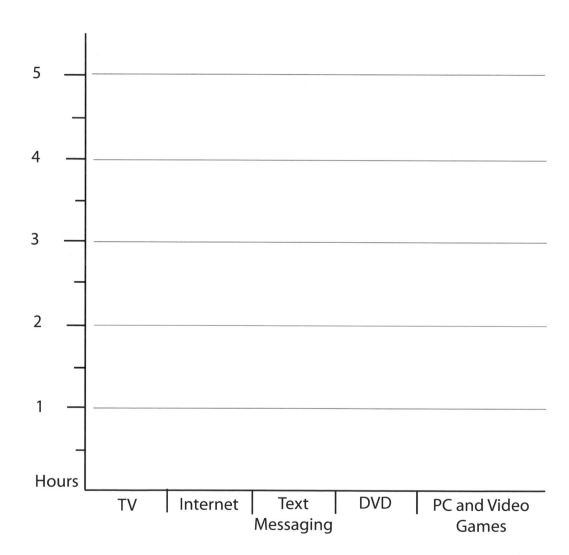

| | TV | Internet | Text Messaging | DVD | PC and Video Games |

5 —

4 —

3 —

2 —

1 —

Hours

Right Now Activity: Instead of Watching TV I Could...

Name: Date:

Make a list of all the fun things you could do instead of watching TV.

Physical Activities	Mental Activities

Now make it happen!

Session 9

Take Away Activity: My Fit Prime Time

Name: Date:

Keep a diary for the week of all the things that you do instead of watching prime time TV.

	4-5pm	5-6pm	6-7pm	7-8pm	8-9pm
Monday					
Tuesday					
Wednesday					
Thursday					
Friday					
Saturday					
Sunday					

Session 10: Media Messages

Resources

Right Now Activity: What's Going On?

Take Away Activity: Media Messages.

Take Away Activity: Something New x 2.

Key Words

Media literacy, products, infiltrate, promote.

Aims

This session aims to:

- introduce the concept of 'media literacy'
- encourage pupils to identify and think about the messages that advertisements and other media messages are trying to get across
- help pupils to become aware of the helpful and unhelpful messages that advertisements may convey.

Review of Previous Session and Take Away Activities

The previous session explored the importance of cutting down on screen time and using this time to get moving and become involved in activities that we can enjoy. Ask pupils for feedback on how they have managed to reduce screen time and get moving since the last session.

Introduction to the Session

This previous session explored the importance of being aware of how much television we watch. Apart from encouraging us to be sedentary, watching TV means that we see lots of adverts. These adverts or media messages infiltrate or have a way of getting into our thinking so that we end up really believing the messages that the adverts convey.

Ask pupils to suggest some of the ways that we receive media messages.

Suggestions may include messages through the following:

- Magazines.
- Newspapers.
- Posters.
- Radio.
- Television.

- Videos.
- Films.
- Music videos.
- The Internet.

Ask pupils why they think adverts exist? Suggestions could be that adverts:

- are trying to sell us something usually ideas or products
- introduce new products
- sell an idea that goes along with the product, for example, if you buy this product you will be cool, attractive, sexy, smooth, rich, successful.

Some adverts bring us helpful information and others adverts provide information that is wrong and encourage us to have unhealthy attitudes and behaviour.

Ask pupils to think of an advert they have seen recently. What was the advert trying to sell? How was it doing this? How did it make them feel?

Take feedback.

Right Now Activity

What's Going On?

Working with a partner and using the advert brought in from home, each pupil should take it in turns to analyse it using the What's Going On? activity page.

Ask pupils to particularly focus on health messages, whether positive or negative, that they think the advertisement is promoting.

Review of Activity

Ask for feedback on the activity.

Take Away Activity

Media Messages

Ask the children to look carefully for all the media messages that are directed at them and choose ten to record on the activity page. They can record the message, where it came from and whether the message was helpful or unhelpful.

Take Away Activity

Can We Trust the Image?

Visit the 'Retouch Website' at http://demo.fb.se/e/girlpower/retouch/

This provides clear examples of how photographs used in advertising are altered or 'retouched'. Check that all pupils have access to the Internet at home. If there are pupils who don't, make time to visit the website with them or suggest that they use their local library.

Take Away Activity

Something New x 2

Remind pupils to keep trying new experiences.

Final Plenary

Reflect and Review

A Circle Time approach can be used to enable pupils to focus on the following:

- Ask pupils to take a few moments to think about what they learned in the session and then suggest a variety of endings for the following sentence, 'One of the things we talked about in the session was the importance of...'.

What Worked Well

- Ask pupils to share with the person next to them something about the session that they have enjoyed. Ask for volunteers to share their responses.

- On a scale of 1-5 (1 = not at all useful, 3 = quite useful, 5 = very useful) how useful do we feel this lesson has been? Ask pupils to do a high five if they thought the lesson was very useful. Ask the remaining pupils to think very carefully about the next question and invite their responses.

- What would we like to be different about this lesson if it was repeated for others in the future?

Right Now Activity: What's Going On?

Name: Date:

Think about your chosen advert and answer the five questions:

1. What is the advert trying to sell you?

2. How is the advert doing this?

3. How does this advert make you feel?

4. Does the advert make you want to buy the product?

5. Is there any health message, either positive or negative in this advert?

Take Away Activity: Media Messages

Name: Date:

Make a list of ten media messages that you receive during the week. Say where the message came from. Think about whether it was a helpful or unhelpful message.

Media Message	From	Helpful or Unhelpful
1.		
2.		
3.		
4.		
5.		
6.		
7.		
8.		
9.		
10.		

Can we trust the image?

Remember to visit http://demo.fb.se/e/girlpower/retouch/

Session 10

Session 11: Everybody's Different

Resources

Right Now Activity: Everybody's Different Bingo.

Take Away Activity: Get Dressed.

Take Away Activity: Something New x 2.

Key Words

Features, complex, diverse, unique.

Aims

This session aims to enable pupils to:

- appreciate that everybody is different

- emphasise that everybody has something unique and valuable to offer

- understand that it is important to value our own and other people's strong points and accept weaker points.

Review of Previous Session and Take Away Activities

The previous session explored how advertisements and other media messages influence us. Ask pupils for feedback on what they have noticed since the previous session about the messages that they receive from the media.

Ask pupils for feedback on their visit to the Retouch Website.

Introduction to the Session

In the previous session we thought about the media messages that we receive through advertisements. Choose a glamorous advert from a magazine or newspaper and show it to the class. Ask pupils to:

- describe what they see

- suggest how the picture may have been digitally altered

- explain what is being advertised

- describe what the person or people in the advert look like

- discuss how the models are selling the product.

Ask pupils to talk through with a partner how they feel when they see advertisements and the pressure that people might feel to look like the images of the people in the adverts.

At the end of this discussion emphasise the reality that humans are complex, diverse and unique and that everybody is different.

In this session we are going to think about all the different things that make up a person. Ask pupils for suggestions and scribe responses under the following headings:

- Physical features and how we look.
- Personality and the sort of person we are.
- Our skills and abilities and the things we are good at.
- Hobbies and interests and the activities we enjoy in our spare time.
- Our beliefs and values.

Right Now Activity

Everybody's Different Bingo

Distribute a copy of the activity page to each pupil. Make sure that each pupil has a pen or pencil. Ask pupils to circulate around the room looking for another person who meets one of criteria on the activity page. Ask the pupil to sign their name in the appropriate box. This activity continues until one pupil has collected a different signature in each of the boxes.

Review of Activity

At the end of this activity emphasise to pupils that there is clearly much more to people than how they look. Ask pupils to think about individuals that they admire and ask for examples. Pupils should be encouraged to think about individuals who have a special talent, the qualities we admire, their achievements, their charity work or the social causes that they support. Pupils may wish to think about the role models they admire within their family, community or among their friendship group.

Take Away Activity

Get Dressed

The activity is designed to make children think about all the factors that influence how we dress (adapted from Chwast, 2012).

Take Away Activity

People to Admire

Ask pupils to visit the following two websites before the next session and identify some heroes that they admire:

1. www.giraffe.org
2. www.myhero.com

Take Away Activity

Something New x 2

Remind pupils that this will be their last opportunity to complete this activity. See if by next week they can savour something different and try a really unusual activity.

Final Plenary

Reflect and Review

A Circle Time approach can be used to enable pupils to focus on the following:

- Ask pupils to take a few moments to think about what they learned in the session and then suggest a variety of endings for the following sentence, 'One of the things we talked about in the session was the importance of...'.

What Worked Well

- Ask pupils to share with the person next to them something about the session that they have enjoyed. Ask for volunteers to share their responses.

- On a scale of 1-5 (1 = not at all useful, 3 = quite useful, 5 = very useful) how useful do we feel this lesson has been? Ask pupils to do a high five if they thought the lesson was very useful. Ask the remaining pupils to think very carefully about the next question and invite their responses.

- What would we like to be different about this lesson if it was repeated for others in the future?

Right Now Activity:
Everybody's Different Bingo

Name: Date:

Find people who:	Signed:
1. Have two sisters.	
2. Love to sing.	
3. Have a birthday in July.	
4. Have a blue coat.	
5. Like to cook scrambled eggs.	
6. Have a younger brother.	
7. Can say hello in three languages.	
8. Have a birthday in December.	
9. Have a dog and a cat.	
10. Have been to Africa.	
11. Belong to a club.	
12. Have been to the local library this month.	

Take Away Activity: Get Dressed

Name: Date:

Think about all the possibilities that influence your choice of clothes. Read the list and tick the boxes that apply to you. Add any possibilities that you can think of. There is a lot more to getting dressed than just how you look.

I dress:			
To keep dry		For breakfast	
To stay warm		To have pockets	
To keep cool		To please my mother	
To be 'cool'		To please my teacher	
To look taller		To be stylish	
For work		To go to a party	
For play		For comfort	
For school		To imitate	
For sleep		For protection	
For sports		For disguise	
For dinner		To cover things up	

People to Admire:

Remember to visit:
www.giraffe.org
www.myhero.com

Session 11

Session 12: Let's Celebrate

Resources

Right Now Activity: Positive Living Skills Dice.

A signed certificate for each pupil.

Key Words

Review key words from the previous sessions as an aid to reviewing the programme.

Aim

This session aims to:

- review the programme and celebrate its completion.

Review of Previous Session and Take Away Activity

Remind pupils that in the previous session we talked about how everybody is different and how it is important to value and celebrate our differences. Did they identify any heroes?

Take feedback on the 'Get Dressed' activity and emphasise to pupils that there is a lot more to getting dressed than how we look.

Spend some time reflecting on the ten weeks of Something New x 2. What were some of the highlights of the savouring and the new activities?

Introduction to the Session

The purpose of this session is to review what the pupils have learned during the programme and to celebrate their achievement.

Ensure that every child is able to articulate the key messages of the programme and know how to make use of them.

Ask pupils to give some of the key messages of the programme. Scribe their responses.

Prompt the class to include the following:

- Eat Healthy Food.
- Get Moving.
- TV Turnoff.
- Everybody's Different.
- SMART Goals.
- Treat treats as Treats.

Right Now Activity

Positive Living Skills Dice

Ask each pupil to make up a positive living skills dice.

Right Now Activity

Circle Time Activity

When the dice are completed each pupil should take it in turns to throw their dice into the centre of the circle and say:

- one thing that they have learned from the programme about the message that lands face up

- one thing that they have put into action.

Ensure that each pupil has a turn to throw their dice.

Final Plenary

Reflect and Review

The final part of the session should take the form of a whole-class discussion aimed at reviewing what has been covered in the programme. Alongside the key messages, it is also anticipated that the children's responses will include their personal views on the usefulness of the programme.

Certificates

The certificates, printed on card and signed by the headteacher and programme facilitator, should be presented to each child individually. It is important that each child knows that their efforts and achievements are valued.

Celebrate

The session should conclude with a small party to include music, healthy snacks and drinks ensuring that there is a celebratory ending to the programme.

Right Now Activity:
Positive Living Skills Dice

Name: Date:

Write a positive living message in each of the boxes.

Try to make up your own positive living messages.

Remember to also look in your log.

The following might help you:

- Eat Healthy Food
- Savouring
- SMART Goals
- Media Messages

- Everybody's Different
- Get Moving
- TV Turnoff
- Treats

Cut out the dice and fold before gluing the tabs and completing the construction.

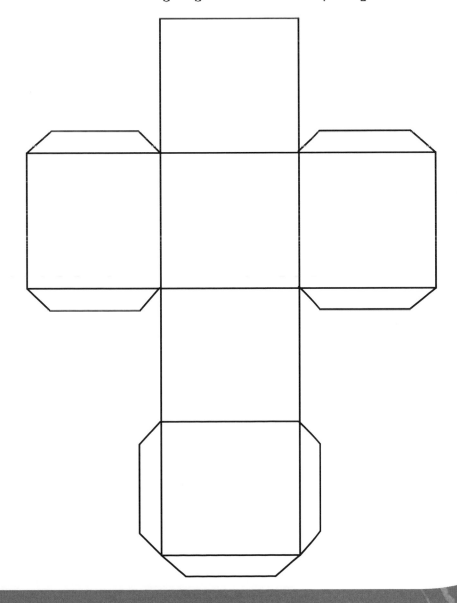

Session 12

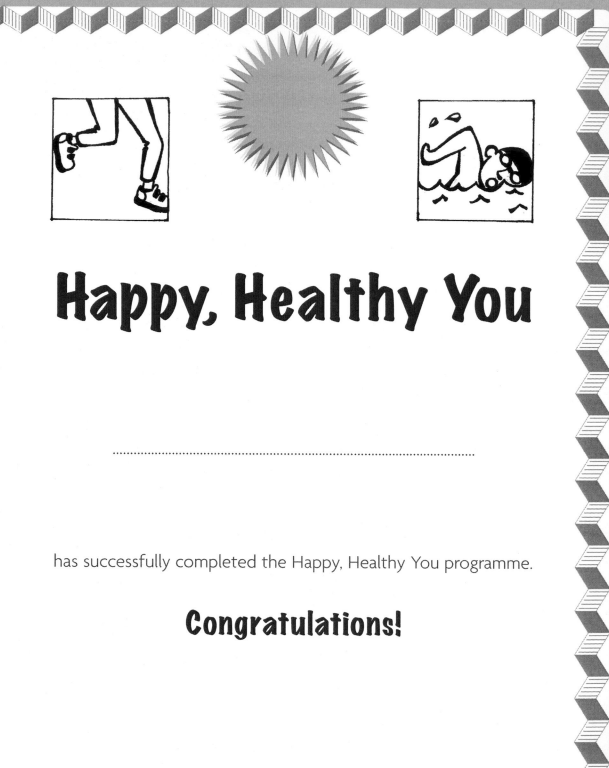

Happy, Healthy You

....

has successfully completed the Happy, Healthy You programme.

Congratulations!

.... Headteacher

.... Programme Leader

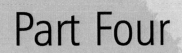

Part Four

Useful Websites and Further Reading

References

Useful Websites

Association for the Study of Obesity.

For detailed statistics and fact sheets relating to the study of obesity.

www.aso.org.uk

Unicef UK has developed curriculum resources on rights and responsibilities for all phases of education.

www.unicef.org.uk/Education/Resources-Overview/

For information on food groups and the serving sizes of food in each food group visit the My Pyramid website.

www.mypyramid.gov

Teaching resources for a healthier, happier life and a child's online BMI checker.

www.mendcentral.org

A fun, educational way to get seven to 11 year-olds up and active.

www.mendmoveit.org

A campaign to encourage all parents and children to make walking to school part of their daily routine.

www.walktoschool.org.uk

Keeping the future fit; the UK's leading, healthy lifestyle activities provider.

www.fitforsport.co.uk

Comprehensive sources of information and links to other websites concerning ways to promote positive body image in people of all ages.

www.bodypositive.com

A website which is all about healthy eating and the simple things children can do to keep fit and healthy.

www.eatlikeachamp.co.uk

One primary school pupil's daily dose of school dinners.

http://neverseconds.blogspot.co.uk

A free one-stop shop for fun nutrition games, healthy interactive tools and fun activities.

www.nourishinteractive.com

Understanding eating disorders and the impact of poor body image.

Helpline: 0845 634 1414

www.b-eat.co.uk

The National Centre for Eating Disorders

54, New Rd, Esher, Surrey, KT10 9NU

01372 469493

www.eating-disorders.org.uk

'Kids and Nutrition' is a constantly revised collection of articles put together to create a one-stop shop for information on maintaining a healthy and nutritious diet for children. It provides a resource for teaching children good and lifelong eating habits.

www.kidsandnutrition.co.uk

A website dedicated to equipping women and girls with the tools to understand and resist harmful media messages that affect self-esteem and body image.

www.about-face.org

Raising Resilient Children is Robert Brooks' and Sam Goldstein's website for teachers and parents. It includes information and strategies for teachers and parents and advertises books and audio materials for sale and has free downloadable information.

www.raisingresilientkids.com

The Giraffe Heroes Project for encouraging today's heroes. This non-profit website honours the risk takers, people who are largely unknown and who have the courage to stick their neck out for the common good.

www.giraffe.org

A website dedicated to celebrating the best of humanity and empowering people to realise their own potential to effect positive change in the world.

www.myhero.com

Further Reading for Children

The following books may give older children an introduction to the subject of childhood obesity. They provide a valuable talking point for parents and teachers who want to explore the issue of fat discrimination with children. Further details on all these books can be found at: www.amazon.co.uk

Cherie Bennett. *Life in the Fat Lane.*

Judy Blume. *Blubber.*

Ian Bone. *Fat Boy Saves the World.*

Chris Crutcher. *Whale Talk.*

Paula Danziger. *The Cat Ate My Gymsuit.*

Barthe DeClements. *Nothing's Fair in the Fifth Grade.*

Louise Fitzhugh. *Nobody's Family is Going to Change.*

Toby Forward and Laura Cornell. *Pie Magic.*

William Golding. *Lord of the Flies.*

Paul Kramer. *Maggie Goes on a Diet.*

Robert Lipsyte. *One Fat Summer.*

Andy Mills and Becky Osborn. *Shapesville.*

Louis Sachar. *Holes.*

Sapphire. *Push.*

J.K. Rowling. *Harry Potter Books.*

Robert K. Smith and Bob Jones. *Jelly Belly.*

Further Reading for Parents and Teachers

Further details on all these books can be found at: www.amazon.co.uk

Ahmad Boachie and Karin Jasper. *A Parent's Guide to Defeating Eating Disorders: Spotting the Stealth Bomber and other Symbolic Approaches.*
Jessica Kingsley Publishers.

Linda Bacon. *Health at Every Size: The Surprising Truth About Your Weight.*
Benbella Books Inc.

Michael Pollan. *Food Rules: An Eater's Manual.*
Penguin Books.

Trevor Dumbleton. *Healthy Eating for Kids.*
Stonham House Publishing.

Jennifer O'Dea and Michael Eriksen. *Childhood Obesity Prevention: International Research, Controversies and Interventions.*
Oxford University Press.

Judith Manson. *Child Obesity: A Parent's Guide.*
Need-2-Know.

Caroline Warbrick. *Eating Disorders and Body Image (Talk About).*
Wayland.

Gary Taubes. *Why We Get Fat and What to do About it.*
A Borzoi Book.

References

Association for the Study of Obesity (2011) *Fact Sheets: Childhood Obesity*, April, 2011. www.aso.org.uk

Bacon, L. (2008) *Health at Every Size: The Surprising Truth about Your Weight*. Dallas, Texas: BenBella Books Inc. www.haesbook.com

Baumeister, R. & Tierney, J. (2012) *Willpower: Rediscovering Our Greatest Strength*. London: Allen Lane.

Baur, L. (2005) 'Childhood Obesity: Practically Invisible', *International Journal of Obesity*. 29, 4, p351-2.

Bayer, A. E. (1984) 'Eating Out of Control: Anorexia and Bulimia in Adolescents', *Child Today*. Nov/Dec. p.7-11.

Bean, R. (1992) *The Four Conditions of Self-Esteem; A New Approach for Elementary and Middle Schools*. Santa Cruz, CA: ETR Associates.

Ben-Shahar, T. (2007) *Happier: Learn the Secrets to Daily Joy and Lasting Fulfilment*. New York: McGraw Hill.

Boutelle, K. N. & Tanofsky-Kraff, M. (2011) 'Treating Targeting Aberrant Eating Patterns in Overweight Youth', in Le Grange D. & Lock, J. (2011), *Eating Disorders in Children and Adolescents: A clinical handbook*. London: The Guildford Press.

Brooks, D. (2011) *The Social Animal: A Story of how Success Happens*. New York: Random House.

Brooks, R. B. & Goldstein, S. (2001) *Raising Resilient Children: Fostering Strength, Hope and Optimism in Your Child*. New York: McGraw Hill.

Bryan, J. (2003) *How can we learn to love our bodies?* www.Channel4.com/health//microsites/0-9/4health/food/abe_image.html

Bryant, F. B. & Veroff, J. (2007) *Savoring: A New Model of Positive Experience*. Mahwak, NJ: Lawrence Erlbaum Associates.

Cavendish, L. (2011) 'But if I eat this will I fit into my jeans?', *The Times*. 29.10. 2011.

Chwast, S. (2012) *Get Dressed!* New York: Abrams Appleseed.

Coopersmith, S. (1967) *The Antecedents of Self-Esteem*. San Francisco: W.H. Freeman.

Corstorphine, E. (2006) 'Changes in Internal States across the Binge-Vomit Cycle in Bulimia Nervosa', *Journal of Nervous and Mental Disorders* 194, No. 6, p446-449.

Csikszentmihalyi, M. (1990) *Flow: The Psychology of Optimal Experience*. New York: HarperCollins Publishers.

Cyrulnik, B. (2009) *Resilience: How Your Inner Strength Can Set You Free from the Past*. London: Penguin.

Dalton, S. (2004) *Our Overweight Children: What Parents, Schools and Communities Can do to Control the Fatness Epidemic*. London: University of California Press.

Department of Health and Department for Education and Skills (2004) *National Service Framework for Children, Young People and Maternity Services*: London.

Faith, M. S., Allison, D. B. & Geliebter, A. (1997) 'Emotional Eating and Obesity: theoretical considerations and practical recommendations', in Le Grange, D. & Lock, J. (2011), *Eating Disorders in Children and Adolescents: A Clinical Handbook*. London: The Guildford Press.

Feldman, S. & Marks, V. (2005) *Panic Nation: Unpicking the Myths we have been Told about Food and Health*. London: John Blake Publishing Ltd.

Field A., Austi, S. B., Striegel-Moore, R., Taylor, C. B., Camargo, C. A., Laird, N. & Colditz, G. (2005) 'Weight Concerns and Weight Control Behaviours of Adolescents and Their Mothers', *Archives of Pediatrics and Adolescent Medicine*, 159, p1121-26.

Foot, J. (2012) *What Makes Us Healthy? The Asset Approach in Practice: Evidence, Action, Evaluation*.
www.janefoot.com

Foot, J. & Hopkins, T. (2010) *A Glass Half-Full: How an Asset Approach can Improve Community Health and Wellbeing*. Warwick, Improvement and Development Agency (IDeA).

Fredrickson, B. (2009) *Positivity: Ground Breaking Research Reveals how to Embrace the Hidden Strengths of Positive Emotions, Overcome Negativity and Thrive*. New York: Crown.

Gill, T. (2007) *No Fear: Growing Up in a Risk Averse Society*. London: Calouste Gulbenkian.

Golding, W. (1954) *Lord of the Flies*. New York: Putnam.

Hill Beuf, A. H. (1990) *Beauty is the Beast: Appearance Impaired Children in America*. Philadelphia: University of Philadelphia Press.

Goleman, D. (2006) *Emotional Intelligence: Why it can Matter More than IQ*. London: Bloomsbury Publishing PLC.

Huppert, F. (2007) *Learning about Happiness, 1st European Conference on Happiness and its Causes*, Conference Workbook, 13th-14th October. London.

Hutchinson, N. & Calland, C. (2011) *Body Image in the Primary School*. Abingdon, Oxon: Routledge.

Kater, J.K. (2005) *Healthy Body Image: Teaching Children to Eat and Love their Bodies Too!* United States, National Eating Disorders Association. www.nationaleatingdisorders.org

Layard, R. & Dunn, J. (2009) *A Good Childhood: Searching for Values in a Competitive Age*. London: Penguin Books.

Le Grange D. & Lock, J. (2011) *Eating Disorders in Children and Adolescents: A Clinical Handbook*. London: The Guildford Press.

Lyons, R. (2011) *Panic on a Plate: How Society Developed an Eating Disorder*. Exeter: Soietas.

Lyubomirsky, S. (2007) *The How of Happiness: A Scientific Approach to Getting the Life You Want*. New York: The Penguin Press.

MacConville, R. (2012) *Building Resilience: A Skills-Based Programme to Support Achievement in Young People*. Milton Keynes: Teach to Inspire, Optimus Education.

Malhotra, A. (2011) 'I Mend Broken Hearts. Then I see my patients being given junk food', *The Observer*, 13.02.2011.

Mann, M., Clemens, M. H., Herman, P. S. & de Vries N. K. (2004) 'Self-esteem in a broad-spectrum approach for mental health promotion', *Health Education Research*, 19, (4), p357-372.

Morbidity and Mortality Weekly Report (2011) Vol. 60, No. 5, *US Department of Health and Human Services, Centers for Disease Control and Prevention*.

Morris, I. (2009) *Teaching Happiness and Wellbeing in Schools*. London: Continuum Books.

National Children's Bureau (NCB) (2011) Highlight No. 250, 'Obesity in Children and Young People', *Library & Information Service*.
www.ncb.org.uk

National Obesity Observatory (2007) quoted in 'British's Power Women are Getting Slimmer', *The Sunday Times*, 24.06.2012.

Nestle, M. (2007) *Food Politics: How the Food Industry Influences Nutrition and Health*. London: University of California Press.

Neumark-Sztainer, D. (2005) *'I'm Like SO Fat!' Helping Your Teen Make Healthy Choices about Eating and Exercise in a Weight Obsessed World*. New York: Guildford Press.

News Review, 'Weighty Issues', *The Sunday Times*, 27.02.11.

O'Dea, J. A. (2006) 'Self-concept, Self-esteem and Body Weight in Adolescent Females: A three year longitudinal study', *Health Psychology*, 11, 4, p599-611.

O'Dea, J. A. (2007) *Everybody's Different: A Positive Approach to Teaching about Health, Puberty, Body Image, Nutrition, Self-Esteem and Obesity Prevention*. Victoria, Australia: ACER Press.

Office for National Statistics (ONS) (2007) *Social Trends*, 37, London.

OnePoll & YoungPoll, quoted in Cavendish, L. (2011) 'But if I eat this will I fit into my jeans?' *The Times*, 29.10.2011.

Parry, L. (2008) 'A Systematic Review of Parental Perception of Overweight Status in Children', *Journal of Ambulatory Care Management*, 31, 3, p253-68.

Pollan, M. (2010) *Food Rules: An Eater's Manual*. London: Penguin Books.

Richards, F. (1950) *Billy Bunter of Greyfriars School*. London: Merlin Books.

Rimm, S. (2004) *Rescuing the Emotional Lives of Overweight Children: What Our Kids Go Through – And How We Can Help*. USA: Rodale Inc.

Roffey, S. (2011) *Changing Behaviour in Schools: Promoting Positive Relationships and Wellbeing*. London: Sage Publications.

Rothblum, E. D. & Solovay, S. (2009) *The Fat Studies Reader*. New York: New York University Press.

Rowling, J.K. (2000) *Harry Potter and the Goblet of Fire*. New York: Scholastic Press.

Ryan, R. M. & Deci, E. L. (2000) 'Self-determination Theory and the Facilitation of Intrinsic Motivation, Social Development and Wellbeing', *American Psychologist*, 55, p68-78.

Segal, J. (1988) 'Teachers Have Enormous Power in Affecting Children's Self-esteem', *Brown University Child Behaviour and Development Letter*, 4, 10: p1-3.

Seligman, M. (2011) *Flourish: A New Understanding of Happiness and Wellbeing and How to Achieve Them*. London: Nicholas Brearley Publishing.

Smith, S. (2008) 'Can we Recognise Obesity Clinically?', *Archives of Disease in Childhood*, 93, 12, p1065-6.

Sothern, M. S., Schumacher, H., von Almen, T. K. & Carlisle, T. K. (2002) 'Committed to Kids: An integrated team approach to weight management in children and adolescents'. *Journal of the American Dietetic Association*, 102, quoted in Dalton, S. (2004), *Our Overweight Children: What Parents, Schools and Communities can do to Control the Fatness Epidemic*. London: University of California Press.

Solovay, S. (2000) *Tipping the Scales of Justice: Fighting Weight-Based Discrimination*. Amherst, New York: Prometheus.

Swinson, J. (2012) *Reflections on Body Image, All Party Parliamentary Group on Body Image*. London: Central YMCA.
www.bodyimage.org.uk

Taubes, G. (2011) *Why We Get Fat and What to Do About It*. New York: Knopf, Borzoi Books.

The Health Survey for England (2007).
www.ic.nhs.uk

Thuen, E. & Bru, E. (2009) 'Are Changes in Students' Perception of the Learning Environment Related to Changes in Emotional and Behavioural Problems?', *School Psychology International*, 30 (2), p115-36.

Weiss, D. (2012) 'Weight Watcher'. *Vogue USA*, April, 2012.

Whitson, S. (2012) *Friendship and Other Weapons: Group Activities to help Young Girls aged 5-11 to Cope with Bullying*. London: Jessica Kingsley Publishing.

Wilson, T. (2011) *Redirect: The Surprising New Science of Psychological Change*. London: Allen Lane.

World Health Organisation (1948) Preamble to the Constitution of the World Health Organisation, as adopted by the International Health Conference, New York, 19-22 June 1946 and entered into force on 7th April 1948.